SUGAR IN MY BOWL

Real Women Write About Real Sex

Edited by

ERICA JONG

ANNIVERSARY
40

An Imprint of HarperCollinsPublishers

HarperCollins books may be purchased for educational, business, or sales promotional use. For information please write: Special Markets Department, HarperCollins Publishers, 10 East 53rd Street, New York, NY 10022.

To contact Erica Jong, please go to www.ericajong.com or www.sugarinmybowl.com, or e-mail to officejongleur@rcn.com.

FIRST EDITION

Designed by Mary Austin Speaker

Library of Congress Cataloging-in-Publication Data

    Sugar in my bowl : real women write about real sex / edited by Erica Jong.—1st ed.

      p. cm.

    ISBN 978-0-06-187576-2 (hardcover)

    ISBN 978-0-06-209220-5 (e-book)

    1. Women—Sexual behavior. 2. Sex. I. Jong, Erica.

HQ29.S84   2011

306.7082—dc22

2011012689

11 12 13 14 15 OV/RRD 10 9 8 7 6 5 4 3 2 1

*For BJG and her brothers
when they grow up*

Tired of bein' lonely, tired of bein' blue,
I wished I had some good man, to tell my troubles to
Seem like the whole world's wrong, since my man's been gone
I need a little sugar in my bowl,
I need a little hot dog, on my roll
I can stand a bit of lovin', oh so bad,
I feel so funny, I feel so sad

—"I NEED A LITTLE SUGAR IN MY BOWL,"
BESSIE SMITH, 1931

CONTENTS

Introduction

W hy are we so fascinated with sex? Probably because such intense feelings are involved—above all, the loss of control. Anything that causes us to lose control intrigues and enthralls. So sex is both alluring and terrifying.

Perhaps that is why assembling this anthology surprised me.

Conventional wisdom tells us that we live in a sex-saturated society where nothing is taboo anymore. Teenagers supposedly give blow jobs at the flash of a zipper. Reliable birth control and Internet mating have made casual sex ubiquitous at younger and younger ages.

So why was it that when I first started asking for contributions to this collection, some women thought they had to check with their husbands before they agreed to contribute? Or their significant others. Or their children, for goodness' sake. (I know that one's children positively *avoid* one's writing—especially if they are literarily inclined themselves.)

I guess I had bought the bullshit that *everything* had changed, that *pudeur* was obsolete, that women today were wild viragos. I knew I had been in a state of palpitating terror about revealing sexual fantasy while writing *Fear of Flying,* but things were supposed to be different now (and I was usually blamed for it).

I was wrong. At least half a dozen contributors to this book would not say yes until their partners agreed.

That was the first surprise.

The next surprise was the fear some potential contributors had that they would not be taken seriously if they wrote for my anthology.

Anaïs Nin had made exactly the same argument in 1971 when I asked her why she allowed her diaries to be bowdlerized for publication: "Women who write about sex are never taken seriously as writers," she said.

"But that's why we must do it, Miss Nin," I countered.

And that *is* why we must do it. We must brave the literary double standard. Doing so, we also liberate our brothers, sons, grandsons, lovers, and husbands—who now write more fiercely and honestly about women—think of David Grossman, John Irving, Jonathan Franzen, and Abraham Verghese—than even Gustave Flaubert, Leo Tolstoy, John Updike, and Philip Roth did in the past.

I admire these men. They can teach a young—or old—writer more about writing than any book purporting to teach the art of fiction. Read them and learn. The ones who came of age after literary censorship gave way in the 1950s and 1960s have plenty to teach.

When did literary censorship become obsolete? It actually happened in the United States within my own memory. I was a graduate student in eighteenth-century English literature at Columbia when suddenly *Fanny Hill, or Memoirs of a Woman of Pleasure* migrated from the locked rare book room to the open shelves at Butler Library. Vladimir Nabokov's *Lolita* was published by Putnam in 1958 after several years of underground notoriety thanks to Olympia Press, Paris. And D. H. Lawrence's *Lady Chatterley's Lover,* first printed in Florence, Italy, in 1928. Henry Miller's *Tropic of Cancer* was first privately published thanks to Obelisk Press in Paris in 1934 and later published in 1961 by Grove Press in the United States.

At first, writers were ecstatic. We thought we would usher in a new age of classical bacchanalia. We thought of Sappho, Aristophanes, Ovid, Juvenal, Chaucer, Shakespeare's bawdy plays, Swift's "unprintable" poems, and of course D. H. Lawrence and Henry

Miller. And it was true that *Couples, Portnoy's Complaint,* and my own *Fear of Flying* promised honesty.

But it didn't take long for *Debbie Does Dallas* to drown out *Ulysses.* Sex, once so literary and rare, got dumbed down like everything else. When published sex became ubiquitous, it also became banal. Profit triumphed over art, and pornography became as dreary as other sleazy products in a culture where everything is for sale.

Many writers began to think it was time to clean up sex. The younger generation—children of hippies and nudists—were, like my daughter, appalled by their parents' freedom.

Why shouldn't they be? Isn't it our job to be appalled by our parents? Isn't it every generation's duty to be dismayed by the previous generation? And to assert that we are different—only to discover later that we are distressingly the same?

Nothing new under the sun. The child is mother to the woman, father to the man. Our parents once were us—and now we are them. Our parents, bless them, thought they were oh so modern.

My own artist/musician parents ran around Provincetown in the 1930s wearing nothing but their scanties (which were much less scanty than scanties are today). They were modern bohemians of the Depression Era. Their children grew up in the fabulous 1950s, when even bohemians could be affluent. And our children grew up in the 1980s, thinking Greed was Good.

Now Depression is back—though we hope not here to stay. But sex hasn't changed all that much. Not since the bonobos and silverback gorillas. We use sex for relaxation. We use it for domination, for power, for pride, for pleasure. We use it to titillate, to ejaculate (including women), to cuddle, and to coo.

We even use it to make babies—although we can use in vitro for that too.

We use it to hold back consciousness of mortality, as Jennifer Weiner's moving story shows. We use it to assert ownership as

Daphne Merkin's story about obsession illustrates. We even use it for love—as Elisa Albert ecstatically shows in "A Fucking Miracle," and we use it to indulge our kinks—as Linda Gray Sexton shows in exploring asphyxiation. We use it to depict outrageous fantasy—as Marisa Acocella Marchetto demonstrates in her imaginative graphic piece, "Cock of My Dreams."

In none of this are we radical. Sappho got there first. And so did Catullus, Ovid, and Petronius, Chaucer, Boccaccio, Shakespeare, Henry Miller, Norman Mailer, and so many others.

We have not invented adultery. Nor have we invented kink. We are just the same old primates who have, for thousands of centuries been hallooing at one another from the trees and doing it behind the bushes.

The beat of blood in the slippery clitoris, the thrusting of the cock—none of it surprises. Fay Weldon talks about her first experience of sex and how much she liked it despite her dowdy mother-made cover-up. She wasn't supposed to like it, but she did anyway. Nature made us that way, and not all the promises of the promise keepers or the purity-ring wearers can change it.

So sex is here to stay—though perhaps not for reproduction—as the prophetic Aldous Huxley predicted.

But we like it. We are made to like it. As long as two halves must come together to make a whole, there is no chance that we will stop clicking the "like" button.

And once women start writing about it, there's no stopping us. *Doing it* is another thing, apparently.

Rereading these contributions, however, I cannot help thinking that the fantasy of perfect sex is far more powerful than explicit sex itself. There is much yearning here, and the yearning is often more thrilling than the consummation. Sexual women are in touch with their fantasy lives. They do not always have to act out their fantasies. I think the so-called sexual revolution misunderstood the importance of fantasy in our lives. We do not have to make fantasy literal to be enriched by it. Fantasy itself is empowering. Because my contributors span the generations, we read about the great range of sexuality—subtle and overt. Sex has changed a lot, and it hasn't. Sex is more about imagination than friction. Most of these efforts are psychological rather than explicit.

I chose to have both fiction and nonfiction pieces because the line between the two has blurred in our time and fantasy enriches both genres. Since *Dubliners* and *Ulysses,* memoir and fiction have drifted together—as Ralph Waldo Emerson and Henry Miller both predicted. And our physical lives cannot be separated from our emotional or artistic lives.

When I asked Daphne Merkin to tell me why she contributed to the anthology, she responded that Freud thought art existed to disturb the sleep of the world. "Anything that prods us into greater awareness, especially of subjects that are blanketed in silence or parody, seems to me to be of use. The sexual arena is so often treated as laughable or minor when in truth it is often serious and major," Merkin said.

I agree. My daughter doesn't—but then she never encountered a locked rare book room.

The mockery and dumbing down of sex in America is something I have often experienced in response to my own books. This is a particularly American response. Europeans do not snicker at nudity or "wardrobe malfunctions." There is probably no other society in which one must argue that sex is an important human drive. Its power is simply taken for granted throughout the world.

Of course sex is allied with death. Perhaps that is part of our discomfort with it. Would we be moved to reproduce if we thought we'd live forever? Probably not. The urge to merge is inextricably joined to our knowledge of mortality. Danger is part of the excitement. That may be why adultery still flourishes and why we are titillated by news of others' adulteries. Risky behavior is thrilling. Walking the tightrope of desire is more spine tingling when the tightrope is stretched over a chasm.

In the end, writing about sex turns out to be just writing about life. There are pieces about childhood sexuality (Anne Roiphe, J. A. K. Andres), pieces about losing virginity (Fay Weldon, Ariel Levy), a fierce short story about sex and illness (Jennifer Weiner), an ecstatic memoir about getting pregnant (Elisa Albert), a tender study of geriatric infatuation (Karen Abbott) and nods to all the stages of life in between. Jann Turner writes about sex and power in her novel excerpt. Rebecca Walker writes about fantasy overwhelming reality. Meghan O'Rourke describes parental secrets and how they mark us.

Barbara Victor writes a short story about sex with the lover her protagonist believes is her last. Honor Moore deliciously contemplates *Story of O*. Eve Ensler writes a dramatic dialogue among women sharing the urgency of sex. Gail Collins responds to the notion of best sex with a hilarious take on the antisexuality of a Catholic education. Jean Hanff Korelitz discusses the paradox of prudishness while writing erotica. Molly Jong-Fast and Julie Klam both confess to the reticence that results from the nakedness of parents, and Susan Cheever celebrates sex with a stranger.

Min Jin Lee awakens us to racism and sexuality. Liz Smith takes us back to Texas sex with kin in the War World II era. Rosemary Daniell chronicles the chaos of sex and alcoholism with an untamed drunken lover. She writes this epilogue at an excruciating moment in her own life. Her son has just died. Susie Bright evokes teenage lust in the era of labor unrest and political protest. Poet Susan Kinsolving writes of mad multicultural love in a satire that reads like poetry. Jessica Winter pokes fun at the scientific approach to sex. And Margot Magowan writes about sex in marriage and its vicissitudes—from vaginal pain after childbirth to a husband's obsession. She also shows how sex and money are horribly linked.

These approaches are as varied as sexuality itself. Happily, there is no way to generalize about them.

The truth is—sex *is* life—no more, no less. As many of these stories demonstrate, it is the life force. If we attempt to wall it off in a special category of its own, we *make* it dirty. By itself, it is far from obscene. It is just a part of life—the part that continues it and makes it bloom.

Like all books, this one has gone through endless metamorphoses. Its working title was *Best Sex I Ever Had* until I realized that books with *Best Sex* in the title were thick on the ground. After trying out *Wild Nights* and discovering that Joyce Carol Oates had used the Emily Dickinson line for a beautiful book of stories about legendary writers, I turned to one of my favorite traditional blues songs. Bessie Smith and Nina Simone both recorded "Sugar in My Bowl," a passionate lament of female desire.

African-American female blues artists were, to my mind, the first American feminist artists to sing of unfettered desire. The honesty of the female blues singer puts much second-wave feminist poetry to shame. The directness of the blues' expression of desire makes the hair stand up on the back of our necks and sends a chill down our spines. This is what poetry is meant to do: tell the truth of human feelings. As one famous blues artist said: "The blues ain't nothing but the facts of life." So the blues have this in common with desire. The blues sing of life in all its rawness and energy. Painful, beautiful, and sad, the blues embrace our humanity without shame.

I hope these fictions, memoirs, and dramatic monologues do the same. There is nothing to be ashamed of in being fully human.

ERICA JONG

A Fucking Miracle

Elisa Albert

I can't say for certain, but I think it happened in Toledo. Late
April, and the weather was glorious. As per usual in Spain, the
vegetarian lunch offerings left much to be desired.

"I hate this," I said, eating my umpteenth olive, eyeing yet
another piece of Manchego, dipping still more white bread in olive
oil. For weeks I'd been subsisting on little else, and I was home-
sick for health food stores, tempeh, vegan bakeries, pleather, like-
minded friends. My beloved tried to ignore me and enjoy his fried
squid. Ham hocks lined the windows and hung from the ceiling,
complete with small plastic cups for carcass-juice runoff.

His silence profoundly bugged me: you love a vegetarian, you at
least fake outrage at vegetarian roadblocks, right?

"Do we really have to have this conversation again?" he wondered aloud, soaking up fish juice with a crust of bread and eyeing
the *jamón* longingly. To his credit, he had abstained from the pig
and listened to my complaints for weeks.

"Should I just pretend I'm psyched about my third bread-and-
cheese meal of the day? My pants don't fit, and I'm not even enjoying the ride."

He sighed.

I might have learned my lesson with my college boyfriend, a midwestern defensive lineman. "I can't believe you expect me to kiss you after you eat that," I once mused, watching him masticate a juicy cheeseburger. He threw the burger away and didn't speak to me for the rest of the night. Why am I fated to love carnivores?

Admittedly, I was being a pain in the ass. Pouting my way out onto the street I went for it, relationship jugular: "You don't care about me."

He stood in silence for a moment before throwing up his hands and stomping away, turning around only briefly.

"*Fuck* you." This from a man so generally kind and even-keeled that the worst I've otherwise heard from him in the way of withering commentary goes something like "S/he means well, but . . ."

I burst into tears, and we spent the rest of the afternoon locked in argument, sitting miserably on a stone path by the side of a church. Clusters of tourists tried not to stare.

Later that night, in our room at the Parador overlooking the city, we made amends. And—wonder of wonders—a baby.

It could, of course, just as well have been a few days later in Madrid, after an afternoon at the Prado, our feet aching. Or a couple of days earlier in Sevilla, flamenco in a tiled courtyard with ivy snaked around the balconies. Or back home in Teruel the following week, in the now-romantic-seeming basement apartment where we spent the spring. Those were busy, amorous weeks, so I'll never know for sure. But I like to think it happened in Toledo. Weary from conflict, overlooking the famous city wherein Jews and Christians and Muslims once enjoyed a golden age of peaceful, productive coexistence, we had ourselves a nice, mature talk and celebrated our mutual love and understanding by getting naked.

We're not an overly contentious pair, though I have been known, for no good reason, to stir shit up on occasion. It's the way things go with us: I am damaged and have issues (see also: "you don't care about me"), he is well adjusted and forbearing (isolated "fuck yous" aside). No, that's not quite right. He has his issues too, but maybe because he's a guy or maybe because his parents aren't divorced or maybe because he's a few years older than I, he keeps things more or less together. Whereas I, often, do not keep things more or less together. Regardless, he is wise and funny and good and humble and steadfast, with twinkly eyes and the body of a swim team captain. His hands are strong, he keeps everything in perspective, he is musical, and he has an enormous vocabulary. Which is to say: I can hardly believe it most of the time—my luck, this ridiculous bounty!—but he is *mine*. When my depressive neuroses bump up against his strong-silent-type stoicism, I am invariably convinced he is going to leave me. When he declines to leave me, much nude rejoicing is in order.

Weeks went by before I knew I was with child ("*Embarazada!*" read the results from the local hospital after I finally realized my irregular period was actually a no-show, went to the *farmacia* for a pee stick, and set out in search of further confirmation), but hindsight is potent, so that night in Toledo has taken on a magical cast.

I know how that sounds. Procreative sex is the height of normative sexual activity, the glory of professional, amateur, religious sexists the world over, and the scourge of the radical feminism that comprised my adolescent imagination. Freedom from it is fundamental to the possibility that a woman can do as she pleases with her life, body, self. It's taken eons to liberate us from reproductive sex, from the notion that sex can only be a means to an end (the end being a *baby,* of course; not an *orgasm*).

I've enjoyed my fair share of unhealthy sexual encounters; there are several last names I can't recall. Suffice it to say that, like the all-too imitable Carrie Bradshaw, I've probably slept with more men than Princess Di but fewer than Madonna. What could be less transgressive than loving consensual heterosexual sex within a committed relationship leading to the exalted birth of a beautiful baby boy? And what fun is sex if it's not at least a little transgressive? But wow: Getting pregnant at that particular moment in time, with that particularly beautiful man, after a stupid quarrel in Toledo, was a fucking miracle. So to speak.

Normally fertile couples have only a 25 percent chance of conceiving at the peak of the cycle. And we—a forty-three-year-old man and a twenty-nine-year-old woman with polycystic ovarian syndrome who'd been fairly malnourished in vegetarian hell—can't really qualify as a normally fertile couple. At fifteen I was matter-of-factly informed by a prick endocrinologist that I'd likely never be able to have children, and I spent the following fifteen years grief-stricken by imagined barrenness, babies the altarpiece of my longing. I screwed my way through my twenties with impunity, using condoms until I knew my partner well enough to eschew them, braced for who-knew-what kind of IVF nightmares. It's chilling to think, now, about all that unprotected sex. I used to joke ruefully about it. The upside of infertility: no worries! If I couldn't be an effortless earth mother, I'd be a husky, world-weary, glamorous sex object instead: forgoing birth control, never staying the night, dragging on a cigarette, beholden only to myself, unfettered by the concerns of regular copulaters. Perhaps I'd shed a lone, picturesque tear for my never-to-be offspring on the subway ride home. Fun was had by all, make no mistake, but I'm blazingly lucky I never found myself facing single motherhood or abortion or STD. I was married for a minute in my early twenties, and the possibility that I might have gotten knocked up then haunts me still: a near miss, stark skid marks in the rearview mirror.

General fertility wisdom holds that a woman is more likely to get pregnant when she's had an orgasm. More blood flow supposedly makes for happier, healthier spermatozoa and egg. And, more to the point, why would nature want us reproducing with a partner who can't make us come? So assuredly we had a *good good* time reaffirming our mutual adoration in Toledo.

We had talked about kids, about when we'd like to start "trying" to have them (code, I imagined, for stressful, routine sex). We thought we might "think about" starting to "think about it" in the months to come. I worried about what "thinking" about "trying" might entail, anticipating a long, hellish road to nowhere. Did we really want to go down that road? Where would that road end? My body wouldn't work properly. Crushing disappointment was inevitable. This narrative became part of my identity, the way I envisioned the trajectory of my existence. I lived with its vaguely sad hum. But fine: I wanted to accept it and move on, preserve our dignity and hormonal imbalances and become one of those fabulous world-traveler couples, resigned to childlessness, nurturing all our nieces and nephews and friends' offspring with joy. Maybe there was an upside to parenting only ourselves, remaining relatively well rested and well ironed. Children were not going to magically appear in my uterus.

We went home to Teruel, the spring wore on, my pants continued not to fit, and I chalked it up to too much bread and cheese, not enough kale and quinoa. It didn't cross my mind that I might be pregnant. I, after all, could not *get* pregnant.

It was early June when I emerged from the bathroom in the basement apartment with the pee stick in my shaking hand. "I'm pregnant," I said, grinning like a lunatic. Then I repeated it, elated and terrified. "I'm *pregnant*," the word a shimmering new planet: glowing, marvelous, and whole, a thing to behold, there all the while. Then he was grinning too, and laughing, and saying *"Really?"*, and we sat on ugly rattan barstools staring at each other, just looking at each other like that, grinning, for I don't know how long.

Astonishingly, unbelievably, there *was* no "trying," no fertility ordeal, no crushing disappointment. Just a good old-fashioned romp with my lover after a quarrel, and now I'm typing one handed while bouncing my sleeping boy in his bouncy chair, singing him a ridiculous song that goes "this is the way we bouncy-bounce, this is the way we bouncy-bounce, this is the way we bouncy-bounce, all the livelong day."

I wanted to give birth at home, under the care of a midwife, away from hospitals and doctors and synthetic narcotics and all the well-documented havoc the above-mentioned are well known to wreak on healthy women birthing healthy babies. I wanted to feel it, to be present, to fulfill the amazing capacity of my amazing body, to experience what giving birth actually *is,* or can be. I wanted, to quote the documentary, an *Orgasmic Birth.*

It. Was. Not. Like. That. Orgasmic, I mean. It was natural, at home, under the care of a midwife, etc. And it was also excruciating and terrifying and lonely and intense and wonderful and awful and amazing and incredible and harrowing. I can't do this, I said, over and over again. And: How does anyone do this? And: I understand why people don't want to do this. *This:* grow a human being inside your body for the better part of a year and then suffer your uterus contracting to push him out through your sex organ.

No orgasm was had. But childbirth *is* like sex, in a way. Or maybe like a hallucinogenic experience, which one can imagine and project and invent endlessly but which, ultimately, can only be experienced as it actually is. There is no imagining, no pretending, and no real understanding to be had after the fact. It is a dream, another world, and then it's over.

With new-mom friends I whisper and giggle about sex, the possibility of sex, like nervous adolescent virgins: Have you done it yet? How was it? How did it feel? What's it *like*? Can I do it? Will it be okay? For me? For him??

Sex is new, and scary, and different, and interesting, and strange. My body has been . . . reorganized. As the amazing Ina May Gaskin, godmother of the modern American midwifery movement, observes: "Men take it for granted that their sexual organs can greatly increase in size and then become small again without being ruined. . . . But obstetricians of earlier generations planted the idea (which is still widely held) that nature cheated women when it came to the tissues of the vagina and perineum (give it one good stretch and it's done for, like a cheap girdle), and a lot of women have bought into the idea that their crotches are made of shoddy goods."

Still, the cliché about how clichés are clichés for good reason is true! This beautiful baby boy is bouncing in his bouncy chair and he fills my mind and heart and arms. Soon he'll be hungry and this brief window for contemplating his conception and birth will be over for now. All I can think is: Love. Love, love, love.

We literally *made love,* a term that until recently I did not like. We made, from pieces of our bodies, from the love we share, a new human being—a love—whose gummy crooked smile and clutching hands and soft skin and shining intent gaze and drunk old man chuckle daily redefine for us the very concept.

I'm glad we're connected in this way: flesh and blood, down to the bone. It's more than married. It's permanent: We were here, this new person is here. There was, is, and will always be a lot of love between us.

My bounty doubled that night in Toledo. (Or Sevilla. Or Madrid. Or Teruel.)

Worst Sex

Gail Collins

When I was a sophomore in high school, a girl in my class got pregnant and had to get married. There were two things about this that puzzled me. One was that her boyfriend, a student at the Catholic boys high school next door to our Catholic girls high school, was the head of a club called "The Beadniks," which was dedicated to finding hip ways to encourage young people to say the daily rosary. Saying the rosary involved fifty-six separate prayers, and even in 1962 we knew there was no hip way to do it.

I decided that the whole make-the-rosary-cool idea had been hatched by a teacher without any student input whatsoever, and that the father-to-be had simply been dragooned into posing as president for the yearbook photo. That sort of thing happened all the time. A nun at my school once decided we needed a club called Students for Decent Styles, whose members would go into department stores, try on dresses with spaghetti straps, and then flounce out of the dressing room while announcing loudly that no decent girl would wear such immodest clothing. I never heard that anybody actually undertook such an expedition; in fact it seemed unlikely that Students for Decent Styles had ever had a meeting. Yet there it was in the yearbook, with a picture of a couple of alleged officers admiring a dress with a very high neckline.

But the really inconceivable part of the Beadniks story was that a girl in my class had been having sex. I was possibly one of the least sophisticated teenagers in the United States outside of Amish country, and although I knew the mechanics of how babies were made, I had not yet really come around to imagining that people actually did that kind of thing voluntarily. (This was at about the same time that the entire universe was talking about the fact that Elizabeth Taylor had ditched her husband to run off with Richard Burton. I told myself that it must all have been a terrible misunderstanding.)

I don't think I was all that untypical, given the time (the prudish early 1960s) and the place (a Catholic high school in Cincinnati). My classmates didn't seem much more savvy. My mother was the kind of parent who would answer any question, and my friends frequently sent me home with queries about sex, which I tossed her way while we were doing the dishes after supper. Many of them, I remember, centered on homosexuality, since we could absolutely not figure out how that worked at all.

This is supposed to be a book about great sexual experiences, and I am very proud that my generation facilitated quite a few such moments during the "sexual revolution" that began later in the decade. But out of pure contrariness I am going to tell you about the staging ground from which we sprang into rebellion, which in my case not only involved no sex whatsoever, but also a long, ferocious campaign on the part of our teachers to keep girls from ever having carnal relations with anyone except our future husbands. Unless of course we chose to join the convent and dedicate ourselves to perpetual chastity.

Really, it's a wonder that we are even functioning, let alone talking about orgasms.

. . .

Until I went off to college, I was taught almost entirely by nuns. This story is going to make them sound a little nuts, but they were in many ways wonderful. They were always enthusiastic, interested in everything we did, and extremely energetic. It was absolutely nothing for them to have classes with forty, fifty, even sixty kids. In grade school, there were so many of us that we were once put on half-day sessions until the parish could throw up a new building to accommodate the early products of the baby boom. My teacher instructed two completely different fourth grades of forty to fifty students, in a room set up in the back of the church. It was a miracle we learned anything at all, but we actually picked up quite a lot. I don't know how strong we were in the specialized areas like geography, where we used a map of the world in which the nations were colored either red (Communist), pink (could fall at any minute), or white (free—for now). Only the United States and Ireland were white. But we got a very good grounding in the basics. The grade school nuns were particularly strong on English grammar. We diagrammed enormous, paragraph-size sentences, conjugated verbs, and separated participles from gerunds with the skill of cowboys moving a balky herd into the proper corrals.

The first school I went to was named after St. Ursula, who went on a pilgrimage with eleven thousand virgins who were set upon by Huns. The way we were told the story, the women were given the choice between surrendering their chastity and being beheaded, and every single one opted for martyrdom. At that point, most of us thought virginity was the same thing as not being married, so I worked up a vague vision of all those Huns rushing toward St. Ursula's pilgrimage swinging swords and brandishing engagement rings.

When my family joined the march to the suburbs, I transferred to St. Antoninus, whose patron was a bishop of Florence in the Middle Ages. He was very learned and had no interesting stories whatsoever. We had an hour's worth of religious instruction every morning, and although it often involved the lives of the saints, Antoninus never came up. Instead, we learned about St. Agnes, who died for the faith when she was only twelve, and St. Catherine of Siena, who was in a hospital tending poor lepers when a mystical vision of Christ so overwhelmed her that she drank the bowl of pus she was carrying. And then there was St. Apollonia, who was the patron saint of dentists because her persecutors yanked out all her teeth before burning her to death. There were, of course, a lot of male saints, too. But except for St. Francis of Assisi (cute animals) and St. Sebastian, whose pictures show his martyred body riddled with so many arrows he could have been a porcupine, the stories I still remember are about the women, most of whom had achieved what the nuns assured us was the highest title a Catholic girl could ever aspire to: Virgin and Martyr.

In high school, we talked much less about martyrs and much more about near occasions of sin, all of which seemed to involve sex.

When I was a freshman, our math teacher had us write letters to Maidenform bra, protesting its "I Dreamed I . . ." ad campaign, in which women were pictured fighting bulls and conducting orchestras, wearing nothing but their bras on top. The problem with the ads, the nuns said, was that they gave boys dirty thoughts. In our letters we avoided discussion of anything so vile, and just claimed that they were an insult to American womanhood, even though the bras in question were serious feats of foundation engineering that covered much more territory than your modern sundress.

That was the same year I went on my first annual retreat, in which a visiting priest urged us to envision Jesus dying on the cross, gazing out into the future, and seeing "you, sinning in the backseat of a car." After that, there were many, many class discussions about how far you could go with a boy before you fell into sin. Non-Catholic boys, we heard, believed that Catholic girls were easy because they could always go to confession and have whatever happened in the backseat forgiven. This was a total misreading of the situation, since I had heard many, many stories about how, on the way home from a tryst at lover's lane, it was possible to be killed in a car crash or murdered by an escaped fiend with a hook for a hand, and be sent directly to hell.

One religion teacher told us that as soon as you started to get sexually excited, it was a mortal sin. This totally undid one of my best friends, who started racing to confession every time she felt nervous or entertained a "bad thought." Eventually her mother sent her to a psychologist, in what was my only experience with a parent interfering in the school lesson plan.

If sinning took place, it was definitely going to be our responsibility. Boys were not much more than little sex robots, and they could not be held responsible for their actions. Once, we were all called to assembly to hear Charles Keating, the head of the Citizens for Decent Literature (and future star of a huge savings-and-loan scandal), who told us the story of a young mother who went walking down the road with her two small children while she was wearing shorts. The sight of her naked legs so overwhelmed a passing motorist that he swerved off the road and killed both the kids. And it was all their mother's fault. We were then asked to sign a pledge never to wear any kind of shorts, including the long Bermuda ones.

There was virtually nothing that happened in the outside world that didn't carry with it some kind of antisex message. When Clark Gable died, our English teacher explained that the reason he had been so successful as an actor was that God, who could see the future, knew Clark would be going to hell for having been married five times. (Since the nuns did not recognize divorce, this meant he had committed adultery with wives two through five.) But he had done some good things in his life, too, and so God in his mercy had given him happiness on this mortal coil to make up for the eternity of torment that was to come. This was my own particular crazy-making moment, and for years afterward every time I got an undeserved A or some other windfall, I fell into a fit of despair over my prospects for eternal damnation.

And so it went. This would be the time for me to recount the moment when I rose up in rebellion, or fell down in the thralls of temptation, but my friends and I really did pretty much stick with the program. I think we were particularly credulous because we were raised in such a sheltered environment—first-generation suburbanites who watched first-generation television programs in which husbands and wives always slept in twin beds. Even my younger sisters, who went to the same schools as I did a decade later, had an entirely different experience. They knew more about sex when they left grammar school than I did when I went off to college.

There are, of course, still Catholic schools today, and I hope the kids who go to them are still diagramming sentences. But otherwise, I doubt they have all that much in common with the ones where I was educated. The girls may wear uniforms, but they certainly aren't required to kneel on the floor each morning so their teachers can make sure the skirts are modest enough so that their hems touch the floor.

I'm sure younger nuns have a much more nuanced view of life and morality than the ones who taught me, but these days there aren't many nuns to begin with. My friends and I were part of the last batch of American women to spend their adolescence being constantly lectured about sex by women who had never had any. My high school had only a handful of lay teachers, all but one of whom were female. The lone male was our drama teacher, who arrived full of plans to produce Shakespeare with an all-girl cast the way the Bard himself did with all men. It broke his heart when he was informed that the school's big annual production was not going to be one of the classics but *The Song of Mary,* which depicted the stories of the best-known recent apparitions of the Blessed Virgin. I was an officer in the drama club, and I got to choose my own part. I picked the girl who kicked St. Bernadette while she was on the ground recovering from her vision.

That was in my senior year, and that particular memory suggests a drift into cynicism that would pick up fast when I got to college and finally figured out what Elizabeth Taylor was up to with Richard Burton. The civil rights and antiwar movements did an excellent job of convincing us that anything anyone in authority said was automatically suspect and that rules were made to be broken. When my friends wanted to start a branch of the antiestablishment vanguard, Students for a Democratic Society, I had no objections as soon as I was assured that SDS didn't stand for Students for Decent Styles.

Peekaboo I See You

Anne Roiphe

His nurse and my nurse were friends. They were both German. His was named Gretchen. Mine was called Geigi, a child's version of Gisele. We lived in the same apartment building. The nurses went to church on Sunday mornings together while we were watched by the cook or maid in one of our apartments. The nurses wore white starched uniforms and no makeup and smelled of soap, while our mothers wore sequins and hats with veils, open-toed Cuban shoes with heels, gold bracelets and ruby rings, and smelled of perfume on those occasions when we saw them.

His name was Jimmy and he loved to draw and he loved me. We were five years old or thereabouts. I had bad dreams and was afraid a witch lived in my closet. He was a little round in the belly and always had paint stains on his fingers, which were blue or red or orange or all of those at once. Our nurses were afraid of germs and taught us to be careful of bathrooms, doorknobs, sneezing children, dirt. Geigi knitted mittens for me. Gretchen knitted scarves. We were at war with Germany. We were Jewish children. The adult world moved around us the way fetid water in a fish tank surrounds the little fish within.

It is raining. The nurses are in the kitchen drinking tea with the back elevator man on his break. We are playing in Jimmy's room. We decide to play doctor. Jimmy has a doctor's kit. We pretend to listen to each other's hearts. Jimmy bandages my thumb. I tap on his stomach. We pretend to examine each other's ears. First he is the patient and then I am the patient. We know how to play together, better perhaps than when we met others later in life. Jimmy draws with his charcoal on my arm. He draws a broken bone and then he sets it and I pretend to cry with pain and he says no, don't cry. I don't like it when you do that. So I stop pretending to cry.

How does a man get you into the bedroom? As many ways as there are men I suppose. How did Jimmy get me into the closet? It's possible I got him. I remember that we went into his closet. I remember the neat rows of shoes, the little folded shirts, a blue jacket with a gold monogram on a small hanger and the cold floor. Jimmy pulled a chair from his small table into the closet, and standing on it he pulled the cord and the light came on. This is the doctor's office he said and now we should take off our clothes so we can examine each other. I remember a feeling of awe and interested fright. I've had that feeling on later occasions: something is about to happen, something good and something worrisome, something that ought not to be but is, something I want but maybe I don't. Something that marks the point where you can't turn back and still keep your claim to sanity.

Jimmy says I have to take my underpants off. I say I will if he will. We have left the doctor's kit on the other side of the door, which Jimmy has firmly closed. I am concerned. I look in the corners of the closet. I see in a shoe an old sock the maid didn't find. I don't see any dragons or other malevolent creatures. We are naked facing each other. I am looking at his face. He is intent, focused, and he is memorizing what he sees. I don't dare look down. I want to look down. I look. I see, for the first time in my life, a penis, a small penis. I see beneath it two small spheres. I see Jimmy looking at me down there. I can't see it he says. You have to lie down. I don't want him to be mad at me. I see my underpants just an arm's reach away. I think about grabbing them but I don't. I lie down. Jimmy kneels over me. Open your legs he says. I need to see. I do. I want to touch it, he says. I know as well as I know my name that Geigi would not approve of this game. She would be angry with me. On the other hand she is not in the closet. She is in the kitchen drinking tea. She will not know. I open my legs. I lift them up and realize I have left on my socks with the little fairies embroidered on the cuff, and Jimmy puts his hand on my wee wee and he leans down to examine it carefully. I feel his hands. I feel the forbiddance of the act. I feel worried but not so worried that I jump to my feet. I lay there as he explored and peered. I think he said there are two holes. Is that right. No I said, just one. He poked with his fingers. I want to look at you too I said and he said all right. It was my turn. He lay down and I bent over him and his little penis lay flat on his thigh and I picked it up gently. I kissed it. Jimmy laughed. I tickled his belly. He jumped to his feet and began to tickle me. We were playing. I said, what do you do with the things below your penis. Nothing he said, they're just there for decoration. Oh, I said. He spit on my chest. I said that's disgusting and I got angry. He said he was sorry and suddenly the door was opened and there was Gretchen and Geigi and one of them shouted put your clothes on. Geigi grabbed me and wouldn't let me pull my own dress over my head but roughly so I knew she was angry pulled it over my ears. A button scratched my cheek on the way down.

Gretchen pulled Jimmy into another room. Geigi slammed the door to Jimmy's apartment behind her and as we were waiting for the elevator she slapped my hand hard. "You," she said, "are a bad girl." "We were just playing doctor," I cried. "Never, never do that again," she said. "All right, I won't," I said.

I lied.

By supper time she had forgiven me. When she brought me my supper on the small tray that I always ate on in my room she sat down on the bed and watched me eat. "When I grow up," I said, "I want to be a doctor." "You can't," she said. "Girls cannot become doctors." "I don't care," I said. "I'll be a patient."

Years later when Jimmy and I were thirteen we were kissing in the dark at a party. We were sitting on a table in my classmates' living room. Couples were curled up together in every corner of the floor, despite the fact that the carpet was rough and scratchy. Louis Armstrong was playing softly in the background. Abandoned in a corner was the Coke bottle that had begun it all. It was a game of spin the bottle that had brought Jimmy and I to the moment. "Do you remember," I said, "when we played doctor." "Yes," he said. "Do you have hair there now?" he asked. "Yes," I said. "I really need to see it," he said. We found a closet. I showed it to him. He showed me his penis, larger, straight penis, full of some mysterious fluid.

No more Gretchen, no more Geigi, just fear of life stopped us from going all the way. But it was good, very good anyway.

The thing about sex is that each act while different from the other even with the same person, even with the same person for forty years, is not a single act. It builds on the sex the night before, the year before, the decade before. Sex is a matter that unfolds like an accordion in the brain, the past is connected to the near past to the present and the future stands there waiting to be attached. So the feelings in the body, the feelings for someone else, the excitement of the new or the welcome of the familiar rises and falls, depends on memory, gains its depth from what happened at the beginning, a while ago, in the imagination, in reality. Jimmy was my beginning and the beginning was fine. Everything after that wasn't always so fine. Sometimes I was scared. Sometimes I found myself with someone I didn't like. Sometimes I wanted to be touched and wasn't and sometimes I was touched and didn't want it. But I think of us in that closet, like Adam and Eve, if God had created them as five year olds. I think of Adam and Eve as poking at each other's navels and laughing.

No one is innocent very long.

Prude

Jean Hanff Korelitz

I am now and I have ever—as in always—been a prude.

I was a prude at age ten, when my older sister told me one of her classmates had a *mattress* in the back of his *van,* on which he had *sex* with his *girlfriend.*

I was a prude at age thirteen, when I discovered that the girls from my bunk at camp were sneaking into the woods with boys, to *make out.*

I was a prude all through high school, reacting with stunned disbelief whenever the rumor of another girl losing her virginity swept down the grapevine, completely scandalized when the class heartthrob (who would later, unsurprisingly, become a performer with an international reputation) "forgot" to put his shirt back on after gym class, and waltzed, half-naked, past my locker. (*Half naked!*) And I was regularly tormented by a classmate who considered my obvious anxiety about sex a source of personal hilarity.

All of this in spite of the fact that my own development wasn't particularly arrested. I freely attest that I played those sweaty, silly games in basements. I had boyfriends and did the expected things with them. I also had sex at seventeen with a boy I really loved (after holding him off for a year). But in spite of all this, my prudishness was of obvious, epic proportions.

What accounts for this?

I haven't the faintest, but I'm not about to waste the opportunity at hand on pointless self-analysis. Nature or nurture—who really cares? And I have bigger fish to fry. I'm here for literary confession and personal catharsis. I'm here to tell that jerk who bullied me in the hallways and the boys I didn't kiss behind the bunk at camp and the guy who forgot to put his shirt back on after gym class and every single person in my life who will be shocked to hear this (in other words, nearly everyone) that there's something about me they don't know.

I am the author of a sex novel.

No, no, I don't mean a novel with sex scenes. I copped to those a long time ago. I'm proud of my four novels, and I'm even proud of the sex scenes they contain, though naturally I can't bear to reread them (they were *painful* to write) and tend to blush horribly whenever people tell me how well written they are.

I am the author of a sex novel. A novel about . . . you know . . . *sex*. A novel in which the sex scenes do not punctuate the narrative but in which the story exists merely to link the sex scenes. A novel you might hide from your kids, as I've hidden my allotted author copies (which I still have, of course—who on earth would I have given them to?) from mine. A novel you might, as it were, read with one hand (which I certainly have not!). A novel I decline, here, to name, by an author (me) whose pseudonym I decline to reveal.

What possessed me? That, as Tevye the Dairyman might say, I can tell you in one word: *frustration*. And not the kind you're imagining. I'm talking professional frustration, career distress. I'm talking mad-as-hell-and-I'm-not-gonna-take-it-anymore dismay of existential proportions.

In 1989, the year I wrote my heretofore secret opus, I was the author of two novels in manuscript that were in the process of being rejected by every publisher on the planet. I had just finished working as an assistant to the editor in chief of an august publishing house, and I had written the novels after work and on the weekends, endlessly tweaking and revising, trying to feel proud of the fact that I was actually, finally creating fiction, something I'd longed to do and been terrified to attempt. When I wasn't writing I compulsively read the novels of recent college graduates (my contemporaries), accounts of young clubbers wasting their time getting wasted, and did my best not to feel cataclysmically jealous. (I was not successful.)

All the while, rejections were arriving regularly, in off-white envelopes with my agent's preprinted return address in an elegant font. It wasn't his fault. I still couldn't believe I had landed this agent, a great guy with an amazing list of writers, some of whom were even published by the august publishing house I'd recently left. I know it hurt him to pass along those letters of rejection, but not nearly as much as it hurt me. As the months passed, the first and then the second manuscript made a slow but inexorable descent from the most elevated publishers to the second tier, down to the interesting paperback imprints and really respected small presses, until there were no more publishers to reject my work.

That's how things stood in the summer of 1989 when I found myself at a tradition-soaked artists' colony in New England, a place where poets and novelists joined visual artists and composers on a campus of splendidly isolated cottages. After breakfast, we would disperse to our cabins for long days of silent creation. Picnic baskets were set gently on each cabin porch at lunchtime, and the cardinal rule was not to approach anyone else's cabin without invitation, lest the interloper disrupt the creation of "Kubla Khan."

I was determined to make the most of this opportunity, and resolved to spend my time revising the second of my two novels, the one that had not yet reached the bottom of its long, excruciating slide down the mountain of potential publishers. That first morning

I dutifully pulled out my poor rejected manuscript, set it before me on the rustic desk, and tried to brace myself for the assault.

I couldn't do it. I just couldn't.

I was bitter about the editors who had briskly dispatched years of my work in letters written by their assistants. I was bewildered and offended by the druggy, barely fictionalized novels, written as senior projects at Bennington, snapped up by publishers for incomprehensible sums, and currently being read by every person on the subway who was not reading *Presumed Innocent* or *Bonfire of the Vanities*. Most of all, I was enraged at myself for spending such a long time writing novels that no one wanted to publish.

I wanted to publish.

I was suddenly determined to use these few, precious weeks to write an entire novel that someone would publish.

I started writing the book—*that* book—that day.

I didn't tell anyone what I was doing. At night, when the other artists blew off steam over dinner and fast games of Ping-Pong in the main lodge, I pretended I had spent the day hunched over my already spent second novel, but my head was spinning with new and very different characters, in altogether different situations (not to mention a vast array of positions). I did not tell my agent about the new book I was writing, because I had no intention of letting him represent it. This book, if it was ever going to be published, was going to be published under a pseudonym.

Ah, the pseudonym! The thinking, feeling, writing woman's armor, time tested and battle worn from its past wearers! Jane Austen went out into the world as "A Lady." Molly Keane, the great girl-chronicler of her horsy, Anglo-Irish set, took her nom de plume, M. J. Farrell, from a pub sign she passed while hacking home from foxhunting, and never emerged as her glorious self until the age of seventy-six, with the publication of her comic masterpiece, *Good Behaviour*. Mary Ann Evans had to become George Eliot. The Brontë sisters all went undercover to write their tales of girls gone wild. Doris Lessing disguised herself in order to see whether her new work was publishable on its own merits or merely because she was Doris Lessing—a fascinating, somewhat depressing experiment for all involved. The book was the extraordinary *Diary of a Good Neighbour* (1983).

I had no such nobility of purpose. I was not defying the sexist literary barricade with one of the few tools at my disposal, nor was I cloaking my identity in order to more witheringly satirize my chums. I was not proving a point, *à la* Lessing, about how publishing stifles new voices in order to spend more money on marquee names. (I should be so lucky as to be a marquee name!) I did it for the worst reason of all. I did it to hide, pure and simple. I did it because the only way I was ever going to be able to write this vividly about sex was to pretend I was someone else, and *never ever tell*. (What, I have always wondered, is the point of an acknowledged pseudonym? Anne Rice wrote the fairly mind-bending erotica under her pseudonym, Anne Rampling, but if she was going to own up to it, why go to the trouble? Her revealed subterfuge seemed, to me, more embarrassing than the erotica itself.)

It's logical to assume that my pseudonym, that firewall between myself and the graphic nature of my subject, performed some sort of freeing alchemy for me as I wrote. After all, *Repressed Female Locates Inner Sensualist Merely by Donning Mask* is a well-worn scenario, but the actual effect wasn't quite so dramatic. My pseudonym did perform this duty only to the extent that it enabled me to get the words on the page; after that, the effect dissipated into nothingness. In my life beyond that novel, even during the actual two weeks it took me to write it, absolutely nothing changed. I might arrive in the colony dining hall each evening after a full day of lips, tongues, organs, and secretions, restraints and responses, but by the time I sat down at the dinner table I had returned to my natural state of unreconstructed prude. (In fact I was appalled at a real life—and very hot—affair between two of the resident artists, one of them married.) And did the thrust (so to speak) of my subject matter at least have an impact on my sex life with my husband? I wouldn't dream of telling you. *Ick! None of your business!*

The truth is that I wouldn't be able to answer that question even if I wanted to, because I don't remember much of anything about those two weeks. I've driven the whole business from my mind. Writing fiction has always been something of an out-of-the-body experience for me, and it isn't at all unusual for me to read a sentence in one of my published novels and not have the slightest memory of having composed it. (I'm convinced that this alchemy of creativity is one reason writers are so fixated on the idea of plagiarism, and why so many interesting stories have been written about shady characters turning up, insisting they are the true author of the prize-winning, bestselling magnum opus, and demanding justice and royalties. Deep down, a part of us suspects that someone else has really written those pages and pages of text, and that we are fraudulently taking credit for them.) When it comes to this particular work, I'm even more at a loss. In fact, every time I try to remember what I was thinking as I wrote those things, those acts, those scenes, all I can come up with is: *What was I thinking?*

Even at the time—and this much I do recall—I had no idea how I was producing this stuff. I hadn't enough sexual fantasies of my own to fill a chapbook, let alone a novel devoted to sex, and though I'd read what might be called the classics of the genre, they weren't much help. *Fanny Hill* seemed too tragic to emulate (enforced prostitution is never a turn-on, no matter how supposedly pleasurable for the prostitute—naturally this book was written by a man), *My Secret Life* too silly to take seriously (likewise written by a man), and *Story of O* lost all appeal for me when the whips and branding irons came out (written, famously, by a woman—*for* a man). Most fortunately, however, I was able to raid the great big public pantry of women's sexual fantasies, thanks to Nancy Friday and her 1973 classic anthology, *My Secret Garden,* a book that provided me with an astonishing range of fictional scenarios. (I didn't have a reference copy in my rustic little cabin in the New England woods, but I had a very good memory.) Friday's feminist approach to women's sexuality was also helpful to me, in that it allowed me to distinguish what I was doing from pornography, which I abhorred. It was deeply important to me that the woman at the center of my story be thoroughly in control physically, emotionally, and financially—the boss of herself, nobody's victim, a person who does exactly what she wants to do for reasons she herself comes to understand only gradually.

To my amazement, the story developed easily, almost effortlessly. Plot had always been hard for me, the weakest link in my two spurned manuscripts, but here, in this book I had neither planned out nor obsessed over, things unfolded naturally. Maybe all the copulating these characters were doing rendered them too relaxed to behave awkwardly. As I made my way into the story, it also became clear to me that, whatever else the novel was becoming, it was also turning into a mystery. This was a surprise of its own. I had certainly not set out to write a mystery. I did not even particularly enjoy reading mysteries. And yet my heroine was becoming murderous before my eyes. Before I knew it, and between set pieces of serious sensuality, she began plotting a perfect crime. Then she carried it out.

And then it was over. To my absolute shock, I had completed a two hundred-odd-page novel in just under two weeks. There it sat, snug in its manuscript box, eyeing me (so to speak). What was I supposed to do with it?

This is what I did with it. I told my husband. He was horrified. I was horrified all over again. But I wanted desperately to publish a book. I wanted to publish a book even more than I wanted to be *known* for having published a book. I promised to keep writing my "real" novels, I told him, but I was going to try to publish this one.

I picked a pseudonym, and I picked an agent, a woman my own age whom I'd met in publishing circles. (Of course, she had to read the manuscript, knowing I was the author—that was hard—but it was also the last time. From the outset I'd decided that people could either read the novel or know I'd written the novel, but not both.) I handed over my box of pages just as I'd handed over my previous novels, then I assumed the usual defensive crouch as I waited to hear from publishers. Always, in the past, ecstatic letters had gone out to my agent, assuring us both that I was gifted and that my work was promising, and then rejecting us both. (I had written these letters myself, in my editorial assistant job, so I recognized them for what they were: simply the approved publishing language and format for "We didn't love it. Good-bye.") But this time there was a different script. A small but respected publisher of erotica liked the book. He bought the book. Then he published the book. In due course, publishers in other countries liked and bought and published the book. And once, a Hollywood producer, who likewise liked the book, decided to make a film out of it. (In retrospect, I'm actually glad this film never materialized.) When my author copies arrived, I promptly hid them, and I never reread or even looked at the novel again. In fact I more or less forgot that it even existed, except when the royalty checks arrived. (Even all these years later, it remains the only one of my books to earn out its advance and pay royalties.)

Years went by, and I wrote other books, which were published under my own name. For these novels my rule became that sex scenes would only occur if they could not possibly be avoided, and perhaps this inescapable quality helped get me over the hump when it came time to write them. Even so, and even given the fact that these scenes were downright tame when compared to my sex novel, I found them harrowing. That was my name on the manuscript, for one thing. And those were my characters, not always lovable but lovingly created. They were whole people whom I'd made, and they were taking their clothes off in public! To get myself through these scenes, I made rules about what could not be said. I would not use clinical language—*penis, vagina, clitoris,* for example, which smelled of the dissection lab. I would not use the kinds of euphemisms that appeared in romance novels and were too silly to take seriously. I would also not use colloquialisms like *cock* or *dick,* which, for me, killed the mood. So what was left? Merely: what the characters, in flagrante delicto, are thinking.

For this approach, which was not, after all, planned, but only a result of eliminating things I was unwilling to say, I realized belatedly that I had an unlikely source to acknowledge. Many years before, I had been vacationing at a seaside resort in Mombasa, Kenya, with my parents and sister, in a hotel filled with people I might now refer to as "Eurotrash," but who at the time seemed to me impossibly sophisticated teenagers. My parents, somewhat uncharacteristically, had allowed my sister and me to attend the evening's social event, a big noisy disco, at which I uncomfortably danced with an older guy from France or Spain or some other exotic place (history does not record this detail). I, naturally, was extremely uncomfortable to be dancing with a stranger in a mostly unbuttoned shirt (Prude!) and more than a little concerned that he would discover I was twelve years old, so I took off when the music ended and went to hide in the bathroom.

Down the hall, in a darkened room, a movie was playing, and I stopped in the open doorway to look. The scene under way was absolutely wanton: an orgy, in fact. I stood dumbfounded in the doorway, watching, and when the setting changed, I went inside and sat down.

The film was *The Seven Minutes,* an adaptation of the novel by Irving Wallace, which I would read a few years later as a teenager. It tells the story of an obscenity trial in California, in which a courageous bookseller faces charges for selling a supposedly licentious novel, also entitled *The Seven Minutes.* The seven minutes in question occur as the Lady Chatterley-esque heroine is in bed with her lover, and the focus of the novel-within-a-novel are the thoughts running through her mind as she is making love. Very little physical description of the act accompanies this stream of consciousness, but the character's very thoughts are enough to drive Wallace's small-minded bureaucrats and PTA types into a collective frenzy. A woman's mind, in other words, is the ultimate sex organ. Fifteen years on, with my unacknowledged erotic novel behind me and the even more daunting task of writing sex scenes for real and complex literary characters before me, I decided that this was the only approach I could possibly take.

This decision, and not my decision to write a novel about sex and publish it under another woman's name, was the catalyst that enabled me to confront this material, and in the years since I have been alternately amused and amazed to find myself called a writer of persuasive erotic scenes. I accept this appraisal. I know I write these scenes well, and not only because I've been told so more times than I can count. I also know because I read the sex scenes in other people's novels, and I find them generally horrendous. (Ironically enough, a long sex scene in Wallace's *The Seven Minutes,* between the hero-attorney and his fiancée, is one of the worst I've ever encountered.) And I know because, well . . . I just know. It may embarrass the hell out of me, but the evidence is clear: when it comes to literary beds, I'm frankly good in them.

Eventually, when the agent with the wonderful list of authors finally dumped me as a client—two novels rejected by everyone on the planet proved too much for him, in the end—I was forced to tell my next agent about my erotic novel I'd published, but thank goodness she never asked to see a copy. Over the years, I confided in one or two friends, always laughing about it, swearing them to secrecy, never once revealing the pseudonym or the title. Once, a British tabloid contacted my husband about a rumor that his wife had written a pornographic novel, and my husband, who was extremely upset, was forced to fend them off. I don't know where the rumor came from, or where it went. And once, in the departure lounge at Heathrow Airport, I was loitering in the Newsagent, trying to find something to buy that exactly fit the handful of English change I had left over, when I happened to look up at the top rack of the bookshelves. This was where they kept erotic novels, paperbacks with scantily clad women and men on their covers. The books had titles like *Hard to Please* and *Everything She Wanted*. One of them was mine. I stared at it. I had never seen this edition. Its cover showed a woman in something that looked like a leather bikini and thigh-high leather boots. She was holding a whip. She appeared extremely annoyed. I bought a copy of my favorite British magazine (*BBC Homes & Antiques*) and returned to my seat, irrationally imagining that the link between myself and the woman with the whip was obvious to all.

So, am I ashamed of what I did? Not exactly. I wrote a novel in two weeks that was pretty well put together, that still pays me royalty checks (albeit very little ones) twenty years later, and—far more important—that gave me the blast of courage that I needed to set aside my two scorned novels (which, as I'm sure you've already guessed, were never to see the light of print) and write a plot-driven book that would be the first of my four published novels (so far!).

So, am I proud of what I did? Not exactly. I still cringe when I remember some of the things in that novel and think about how horrified I would be if someone who knew I had written it actually read it. Because, although I am the twenty-years-married author of an erotic novel (not to mention racy scenes in my acknowledged novels), I am still, as I always shall be, the most straightlaced person I know.

A few years ago I had a sadly telling conversation with my friend Elisa. We were talking about *Sex and the City,* and I was taking issue with the morning-after debriefings those characters enjoyed, the free and open discussion of sexual foibles, triumphs, and predicaments. I didn't believe that for a second. "It's ridiculous, the way they talk about sex," I told her. "I mean, I wouldn't dream of talking to my friends about my sex life. It's so personal. Men do that, I guess, but women just don't discuss sex."

"Jean," Elisa said, sighing, "I talk about sex with *all* my friends. Except for you, of course. You know, you're such a *prude.*"

Sex with a Stranger

Susan Cheever

Growing up in the 1950s, I heard many stern warnings about one-night stands. Men don't respect you afterward. They won't buy the cow if they can get the milk for free. Personally, I don't like being compared to a cow. Furthermore, stern warnings often inspire me to do the opposite of what I am told. Maybe that's why I've always loved one-night stands.

I never was one for picking up men in bars or in the next seat on an airplane. I usually met them at parties—New York is a city of parties. The two of us would start to chat, and the chat would become something more serious. We talked about work and our ambitions. We'd find a common interest in Edith Wharton or the Boston Red Sox. Soon we were sitting somewhere private in a corner. We would have another scotch or another glass of wine.

Then we would begin to touch each other—a hand on a shoulder to make a point, a light squeeze of the knee if a joke was particularly funny. I felt that familiar hot and cold feeling, that soaring and sinking, which I knew was my mind being overwhelmed by my physical excitement. I let it happen. Sometimes we would leave for a drink at a neighborhood bar; sometimes we simply took a taxi back to my apartment. In the cab, we kissed. I wondered about the condition of my apartment—had I made the bed? We kissed again and I forgot about housekeeping. Soon, we would be in my unmade bed, embracing each other and experiencing the awkward, thrilling moments of sex with a stranger.

If you are looking for love, sexual intimacy can be a shortcut. It is among the fastest ways to get to know another person. During sex, we literally and figuratively expose ourselves. We show physical parts that are usually kept covered; we display our private likes and dislikes. In its moments of unconscious response to physical pleasure, the body reveals a great deal of information: a need to dominate, a difficulty following suggestions, an inability to express desires. If we have trouble letting go or if we are painfully uncomfortable with how we look, it often shows up in the two-person drama of the sex act.

It's scary to do something that lets another person in on so much private information, so many fears and discomforts, but it's also ruthlessly efficient. Dinner in a fancy restaurant or even a long conversation in a dimly lit bar can be completely misleading. In e-mails and letters and telephone calls, people can act their way into being someone different. It's easy to fool someone with a turn of phrase. Sex tells the truth.

Most erotic fantasies are about one-night stands. In my own, I imagine having sex with someone I've started dancing with at a party. We end up in a bedroom on a pile of coats left there by other partygoers. I smell the scent of someone's perfumed lining and feel the softness of mink against my naked legs.

Somehow, I never fantasize about sex with my husband in a marital double bed that I've neatly made with hospital corners, or with a man who has just changed our baby's diapers or emptied the dishwasher. Marriage can be sexy, too, but in my experience, it is never the stuff of fantasy. I think this is nature's way of telling us that sexual intimacy is distinct from emotional and financial and domestic intimacy. What's wonderful in bed can be disastrous in the nursery or the kitchen.

My deepest connections to men have often been at times when sex seemed like an impossibility, or at least an unpleasant after-thought. Two weeks after the birth of my beloved son, his father went to my favorite lingerie store and bought me a fabulous black lace teddy. I oohed and aahed politely as I unwrapped the layers of pink tissue, but the truth was that the skimpy fabric looked like an artifact from another life. Childbirth and its aftermath had given me enough discomfort for a lifetime. I could no longer imagine why a woman would ever wear such an impractical thing.

When my husband and I finally did have sex after the baby was born, it was without the seductions of black lace. It was clumsy. Ten-tative. It felt like sex between two people who had just had their first conversation. It was, in many ways, like a one-night stand.

When I was a young woman in the early 1960s, I knew my life wouldn't really start until I was married. Abortion was illegal, and we all knew horror stories about what could happen to women who tried it anyway. Birth control was unwieldy and difficult to get—a visit to Planned Parenthood with a fake engagement ring one after-noon yielded me nothing but embarrassment. Given the situation, I planned to sleep only with men who were willing to marry me. The trouble is, my sexual enthusiasm far outweighed my desire to be a twenty-year-old housewife. Still, I managed to restrain myself: By the time I did get married at what I thought was the ripe old age of twenty-three, I'd been sexually intimate with only a few men I'd assumed I would be with for the long haul. What we think of as the swinging 1960s didn't really begin until the early 1970s, and it wasn't until the sad end of my first marriage that I was released into the wild, fevered sexual freedom of that time. By then, abortion was legal and birth control was available and easy to take. No one had heard of AIDS.

A one-night stand is the erotic manifestation of carpe diem—only we are seizing the night instead of the day. Though sex with a long-term partner is many things, it is not that. With a husband or a boyfriend, there is the delicious certainty that pleasure will be both given and received. Sex feels like a series of shared secrets, a passage through a maze leading to the most wonderful feelings available to human beings. With a long-term partner, I can relax. He is not surprised by the moles on my back, nor is he self-conscious about the hair on his shoulders. There's a kind of transcendence to married sex, a connection that is more than the sum of body parts linked and flesh responding, as if this most physical of acts was also the threshold to spiritual intimacy.

One-night stands can be spiritual in another way: they can be sex without expectations. They are a leap of faith because you never know quite where they will lead. My one-night stands were never planned, and they were always, in their own ways, mysterious. Occasionally they took place in the afternoon in a hotel. Once, there was a dazzling ten-minute interlude bent over a washing machine with a fellow Sunday luncheon guest in someone else's suburban laundry room. When I was an editor at *Newsweek,* they sometimes happened early in the morning in the little infirmary room next to the copy machine. At the time, staying at the office until the next morning and editing in the same clothes was a rite of passage for anyone with ambition. One night, a writer I admired was also working late, and we ended up walking out of the lobby together and into the romantic early-morning streets. Remember Marlon Brando singing about that time of day in *Guys and Dolls*? "The street belonged to the cop, and the janitor with the mop . . ." The writer offered to see me home.

When we got there, I opened a bottle of wine. "Let's drink this in bed," he said. Afterward, we both fell asleep for a few hours, and I woke up thinking about how much happier I'd be if he wasn't there.

I admired his work, not his body. He snored. He took up a lot of space in my bed. When he finally roused himself, he halfheartedly asked if I wanted to go out for breakfast, and I pleaded a headache. After that, we went back to being friendly office mates. We had tried out a different kind of relationship and found that it didn't work.

One-night stands can be nothing more than a few hours of pleasure, or they can be the beginning of something much more important, and it's impossible to tell until it's too late. Another man I slept with, never intending anything serious, was married to an acquaintance of mine, but she was far away. It was summer in New York City, when wives and children stayed in the country and all domestic rules seemed breakable. It was too hot to feel guilty as I should have felt. Slowly, with a lot of laughter and in the kind of emotionally woozy state that results from staying up too long, we repaired to my bedroom. The sex wasn't particularly memorable; we were both tired and quite drunk. I fell into a fitful sleep and woke to find myself sheltered in his arms. His flesh was pleasantly warm. He smelled good. I drifted off again, feeling buoyant and safe.

When we officially woke up a few hours later we tried to pretend that everything was normal. I made coffee and changed the sheets. He got on the telephone with an editor, then called his wife and checked on his children. It was no use. By the time we wandered out to lunch we both knew something huge had happened. Our connection felt capricious, as if there had been a potion in my nightcap, or as if a rascally little boy had aimed an arrow in our direction. We sat in a bar, holding hands, reveling in our exhilaration at having found each other and in our suffering at having to part. It was as if we had been together forever; I felt an uncanny sense of destiny fulfilled. The world, however, didn't care. I had to be in Boston for dinner. He had a plane to catch.

That one-night stand led to a thirty-five-year love affair—the most enduring love of my life. Some kind of deep intimacy between us had been released, an intimacy that remains decades later. After more than fifteen years of obstacles—my guilt, his guilt and pain, limited resources, our own confusion—we eventually married and had a wonderful son. I had no idea what was going to happen when I casually invited him up to my apartment. If I had known, would I have gone home alone?

That is the real danger of a one-night stand. Not that it will lead to nothing, but that it will lead to everything. In this way, casual sex is excruciatingly hazardous. Those who are not ready to have their life changed should probably abstain.

Everything Must Go

A Short Story

Jennifer Weiner

The twins were almost ten months old when Lizzie found the lump. She hadn't been looking for it, she hadn't been doing a self-exam, she had simply been standing, immobilized, underneath the pounding water, more asleep then awake.

When Cal came into the bathroom, a towel knotted around his midsection, she blushed like a kid caught cheating, reached for the soap and started soaping herself vigorously, turning her back toward her husband, so that he wouldn't catch a glimpse of her slack, stretch-marked flesh. Lifting her breasts to wash beneath them, her fingers chanced against the lump, skated over it, then returned again, her skin going instantly icy beneath the warm water.

She stepped out of the shower with soap still slicked on her body. Cal was peering in the mirror, smoothing shaving cream over his cheeks, and one of the twins (her money was on Logan) was wailing from his ExerSaucer outside the bathroom door.

"You're dripping," he told her.

"What's this?" she said, and grabbed his hand. His razor clattered in the sink.

"What's what?" Cal looked annoyed. Cal frequently looked annoyed these days. It was the babies, the sleepless nights, the messy house, her own preoccupation. Plus, he was working so hard, doing whatever he did in his suits, at his office downtown (she'd once known every detail of his day, back when she'd worn suits and had an office of her own).

"What's what?" he asked again. "Look, Lizzer, I've got an eight o'clock . . ."

She lifted his fingers to the place where she'd felt the lump and pressed, keeping her eyes on his face. "There's something there, right?"

His fingers probed briefly, then withdrew. "It's probably a milk duct," he said, and picked up his razor again.

"It's not," she said, hearing panic in her voice. "This feels different."

"So have Lemmin take a look." He drew the razor over his boyish face in smooth, unhurried strokes, and at that moment, she could have easily snatched the blade from his hand and slashed his throat.

The radiology department was in the hospital's basement, and it was, predictably, dark, but someone had made an effort with potted hydrangeas, brilliantly blue, and a tank full of darting beta fish. Lizzie sat, topless, goose-bumped, her breasts compressed between clear panes of glass, thinking ruefully that this was the most time she'd had to herself since the twins had come.

Back in the waiting room, idly flipping through a limp issue of *People,* she jumped when the nurse tapped her shoulder. *Nothing to be alarmed about . . . a common procedure . . . just double-checking.*

The needle was so fine she barely felt it go in. Ten minutes later, she was out into the sunlight with a Band-Aid on the side of her breast. After fighting traffic on the Schuylkill for forty-five minutes, she arrived home to a sink full of dishes and two screaming, overtired boys, a sitter (a little rat-faced girl who Lizzie just bet would be pregnant before she finished high school) demanding eighty dollars, and a husband who rolled in at eight o'clock (after the baths, after the stories, after twenty minutes of nursing and two diaper changes), cast a cool eye over the cluttered counters and the floor dotted with rotini and peas, and said, "No dinner, huh?" and didn't even ask how her appointment had gone.

Dr. Lemmin called the next morning. From his tone when he asked,"Can you stop by the office?" from the way he asked whether Cal could come, too, she knew that the news wasn't good. "I'm so sorry," he said.

Sitting there, stunned and numb, in the same chair where she'd sat when he'd told her she was having twins, Lizzie didn't listen, hadn't made out anything since he'd said *cancer*. The words washed over her like the water in the shower. "If it were you," Cal's voice interrupted, high and whiny, like a mosquito she wanted to swat. "If it were your wife . . ."

The doctor didn't hesitate. Double mastectomy. Lymph nodes, ovaries, and uterus. The whole shooting match. Numbly, Lizzie had nodded. "That's what I want," she'd said, and when Cal interrupted, said something about considering their options and second opinions, she'd cut him off, her voice shrill and peremptory. *That's what I want. Everything must go.*

Three days later, at six in the morning, she rolled over, and announced, "I'm going shopping." Beside her in bed, Cal merely nodded. Her husband, normally so tanned, rosy-cheeked, and cheery, looked pale and shell-shocked, his face slack and jowly, his eyes wet and wounded, as if, she thought meanly, cancer was something she'd gotten just to upset him.

"On Thursday, I'm going shopping in New York," she said. "For the day. Maybe I'll stay over." He nodded again. He set one hand on her shoulder, lightly, then lifted it off, as if her skin burned.

"Whatever you want," he said. He paused, and she could tell he was waiting for something. For what? For her to thank him? For her to say "I love you"?

She squeezed her eyes shut, saying nothing, holding still even after she heard the boys start to coo, then fuss. After a minute, Cal went to them. She lay there, listening as he struggled to diaper and dress them, and then carried them, one at a time, into the kitchen, where he made a noisy show of doling out bananas and Cheerios.

Lizzie pulled her iPhone out from underneath the pillow where she'd stashed it the night before, and tapped in an e-mail address she'd looked up the night before, writing, in the memo line, *Is this you?*

Seven minutes later, her in-box pinged.

IT'S ME. WHAT'S UP, KID?

Recklessly, breathing hard, face flushed, fingers scrabbling at the tiny keyboard, she typed out:

I'VE BEEN THINKING ABOUT YOU. GOING TO BE IN YOUR NECK OF THE WOODS ON THURSDAY. ARE YOU FREE?

It took him nine minutes this time.

YOU TWISTED MY ARM. TELL ME WHERE AND WHEN.

You're not really doing this, are you?

The question teased at the back of her mind as she made her calls, scheduling the port insertion, Googling support groups and nutritionists, setting up the first round of chemo, scheduling the operation. "Maybe I'll be a B cup," she'd joked to the unsmiling surgeon. "You know. Perky."

Lizzie had never been perky. She'd been a double D in eighth grade, and hadn't that been a picnic, and she'd only gotten bigger since having the boys. Her breasts made shopping a misery, had guaranteed hoots and whistles from every construction site she'd ever had the misfortune of passing, had ensured that every dress she bought required alteration, and that breast-feeding was more of a workout than some women got at the gym. Her breasts were an encumbrance, an embarrassment, and she'd planned, once the boys were done nursing, on having them reduced.

Cal liked her breasts just fine, although she'd accused him, more than once, of treating them like cantaloupes he wasn't sure he'd wanted to buy, but Marcus, the last boyfriend she'd had before her husband and the one she still thought of, especially after a glass or two of wine, as the love of her life, had adored them.

In bed with him, for the first time, he'd reverently unfastened the clasps of her bra, and then sighed, like a man glimpsing heaven, when her breasts had tumbled into his hands. He had caressed them gently, then firmly, working at her nipples with tongue and teeth until Lizzie would be tossing her head and shuddering against him. Sometimes he'd slick them with lotion and straddle her body, cupping her breasts against himself, rocking back and forth in the slick channel they created until he threw back his head, handsome features contorted, groaning, spurting over her chest and her cheeks.

Oh, Marcus had loved her breasts. He'd loved her, too—maybe, she thought sometimes, better than Cal did . . . but Marcus, tall and fair and slim where her husband was short and curly-haired and boyish, was twelve years older than she was and already divorced when they'd met, and he'd made it abundantly clear from the beginning that he wasn't the marrying kind. When she was twenty-eight, after three years together, Lizzie had broken up with him. She'd moved out of their apartment and spent a month weeping, unable to eat. Then, eleven pounds thinner and with shadows under her eyes and interesting hollows under her cheeks, she'd posted a picture online and spent the next two years dating anyone who'd asked. It had been two years of bad dates, and blind dates, and Jdates. And then she'd met Cal.

For the last ten years she'd been happy . . . or, at least, she'd thought she had. If her sex life with Cal wasn't as torrid as it had been at the beginning (and if, even at the beginning, it was never as torrid as it had been with Marcus), well, then that struck her as an acceptable trade-off for all of the other things she'd wanted, and gotten: the house in the suburbs with the excellent public schools, the children who would one day attend them, the SUV with four-sided air bags, the two weeks at the shore in August and the ten days in the Keys over Christmas; a man who'd promised to love her forever, who'd share popcorn at the movies and kiss her on New Year's Eve. She'd thought that was enough . . . only now, she wasn't sure.

Cal came back into the bedroom and kissed her. "Love you," he whispered and went to work. When the sitter arrived, Lizzie locked her bedroom door, went online, and booked a room at the Plaza. Eight hundred and fifty dollars. The total took her breath away. *It's just dinner,* she told herself, tapping in the credit card number. Just dinner with an old friend. And don't I deserve something nice? After all these months, after all this sleeplessness and sexlessness and now cancer, motherfucking cancer, don't I deserve a treat?

Her suitcase looked as if it had been packed by a crazy person. A lacy black thong lay on top of a pair of stained cotton briefs. A matching black bra, with a tiny rosebud sewed between the cups, was tucked beneath a sturdy beige nursing bra. Strappy black sandals (will!) danced on top of black clogs, the right one with a splotch of YoBaby yogurt over the toes (won't!). Lizzie tossed in her best dress, the one made of fine black wool, with the plunging neckline, and dug through her jewelry box to find her diamond necklace, a solitaire suspended on a platinum chain, that Cal had given her when the boys were born. She fastened the clasp, zipped up the suitcase, waved to the sitter, and dashed out the door before the boys could notice she was gone.

"Very good, madam," the bellhop approved, unlocking the door to her room, as if Lizzie's jeans and flats and Eileen Fisher tunic were the finest things he'd seen all day. Black-suited, white-gloved, he bustled around her room, opening the curtains, demonstrating how the television could be made to rise from its enclosure at the foot of the bed, adjusting the temperature, bringing her ice. She tipped him twenty dollars, eliciting a second, even more enthusiastic "Very good," and when he was gone, she lay on the bed, staring up at the crown moldings, with her bare feet on the crisp coverlet, and her hands resting lightly on her breasts.

She slept, then ordered high tea from room service, nibbled at the salmon and egg-and-cress sandwiches before carrying the glass of Champagne into the bathroom, where she took a long, hot bath. She lathered her body with creamy soap. She shaved her legs and smoothed on lotion, and wriggled into her lacy underwear, then the high-waisted spandex boy-shorts that left her breathless and made it look like she was roughly the same size she'd been, prebabies. Downstairs, at the bar, she ordered a glass of Riesling, and sat on a stool, legs crossed, heart pounding, until she felt his hand on her shoulder and heard the low rumble of his voice in her ear.

"Elizabeth," said Marcus. She'd always been Elizabeth to him, never Lizzie, never Betsy or Beth. He said her name and hugged her awkwardly, one armed, as she half-rose from the barstool, and it was as if nothing longer than a three-day weekend had passed between them, as if she'd woken up that morning in his bed and murmured *Hi, handsome* into his neck.

"Hi, handsome," she'd said reflexively, and he'd smiled, flashing his teeth. Immediately, she felt the physical response to his voice, his touch, his body, his dear, familiar scent and wondered if it was meant to be as simple as that—you picked the one who smelled right to you (Cal, she thought, before she could stop herself, smelled like breath mints and Right Guard, which wasn't nearly as nice). As always, she felt his voice right between her legs, as intimate as if he'd reached down and cupped her there.

Her knees wobbled as she stood. "Whoops," he said, and took her hand, her right one, the one without the wedding band, and led her into the elegant restaurant, all plush carpet and velvet banquettes and not a high chair, or a child, in sight.

They ordered from a menu full of delicious-sounding dishes, although, later, Lizzie couldn't have said how any of it tasted—there was pâté, a chilled soup, duck with white peaches and skate wing braised in brown butter. Marcus ordered white wine to start with, then glasses of red, a spicy Rioja. He talked amusingly about his job as a corporate litigator—the crazy hours, the crazier clients—and Lizzie talked about her kids. Over port and cheese and walnuts, he asked, "Are you happy?" and she'd shrugged, lowering her eyes, saying, "Well, it's hard."

"It's a good thing you're doing." He leaned forward, pale eyes intent. Lizzie nodded. It had taken her a long time and many sleepless nights to figure that out—that it truly wasn't her, but him; it wasn't that Marcus didn't want to marry her, it was that Marcus, damaged by his own childhood, his own ruinous first marriage, didn't want to marry anyone.

When she looked up again she saw that the restaurant was empty, the waiters hovering politely around the perimeter. Marcus insisted on paying and walked her to the elevator. There, on the tiled floor, beneath a dazzling chandelier, he took her in his arms and held her closer than was technically proper. "Elizabeth."

She let herself relax in his arms. *Will. Won't.* Marcus sighed. She felt his lips graze the side of her neck, but she knew that he wouldn't push it, that it was up to her. Her call. Her move.

Lizzie tilted forward, pressing her breasts against his chest. She twined her arms around his neck, and rose on tiptoe, her lips brushing his ear. "Want to come up with me?" she whispered, and he hesitated for just an instant before he said, "Okay."

The elevator doors slid open. They stepped into the mirrored chamber . . . and then Lizzie was in his arms, her hips pressing against his, and his tongue was in her mouth and his hands were on her breasts, molding them, caressing them, sighing, as if he'd been starving and now, finally, he had food.

The doors opened. Hand in hand, they hurried down the hallway. In the room, the bed was turned down, the television set standing proudly erect, having emerged from the sheath of its case. "It wasn't like that when I left," Lizzie said, and Marcus laughed. She closed her eyes, overcome, as the sound of it rippling through her.

Then they tumbled onto the bed, and there, rolling on the covers, with his mouth, hot and insistent, over hers, she was twenty-five again, twenty-five and just meeting a tall, sleekly blond attorney who'd slid a martini, her first martini, on the bar in front of her and said, *Try this, you'll like it.* Two hours later, she'd gone home with him. She'd been in grad school, and he'd been out with friends, and she'd never done that, never met a guy in a bar and slept with him that same night, not before and not after.

On the hotel bed, Lizzie closed her eyes, running her hands down the smooth length of his back, hearing herself make sounds she hadn't made since labor. *Just this,* she thought. *Just kissing.* Just this is all the sweetness I need to hold me, to get me through what's coming . . . plus, he's fifty. Maybe he can't anymore. But then Marcus lay on top of her, and it was very evident that, even at fifty, he could.

He bent his bright head to her breasts. She felt his tongue working against her, and wondered if he sucked, whether there would be milk, and how it would taste. *I love you,* she thought, astonished at the sweetness of it, pulsing through her with her heartbeat. *I'll always love you.* She felt him poised against her, breathing hard and trembling, the tip of his cock hot and slick but waiting, again, for it to be her choice. Lizzie twisted her hips and felt him slip inside of her.

Afterward, lying spent and flushed beside him, she said, *That was lovely,* and he smiled lazily, one hand still between her legs, saying, *I want to watch you come again.*

At three in the morning, when one or the other of the twins usually woke up, she pulled the crisp white cover up to his chin, and bent to deposit a gentle kiss between his shoulder blades.

At six, he woke up, drew her against him. *Oh, baby,* he groaned, his mouth hot against her breast where, until that morning, the bandage had been, and she felt her throat close. *I should tell you,* she started to say. *Tell me what?* he asked, and she shook her head, swallowing the words *I'm sick, I'm having an operation, I won't have breasts at all next week.* Instead, she pressed her lips against his and straddled him, slipping him inside of her and riding him, with her breasts dangling over his lips like ripe fruit, like the grapes Tantalus could never quite reach.

Later, with her body twined around his, she said, *I love you,* and he said, *Love you too, kid,* tears slipping from his eyes because, of the two of them, he'd always been quicker to cry . . . and quicker to sleep.

For a few rapturous moments, Lizzie rested her cheek on her hand and watched him breathe. Then, when pearly grayish light was filtering through the blinds and the city was starting to wake beneath her, she slipped out of bed, gathered her clothes from the floor, and bundled them into her suitcase.

She left the maid twenty dollars. She left Marcus a note. *This was perfect. I love you. xx, E.* Then she pulled on her mommy uniform, tugged her suitcase behind her, and eased the door open, then shut.

Love Rollercoaster 1975

Susie Bright

I cut last period, high school driver's ed with Mr. Gorshbach. He wouldn't understand that the revolution was not going to wait for me to take his stop-signal exam. Instead, I grabbed the bus and showed up at Gateway Freight yard right before the start of swing shift like I promised I would.

I changed my clothes too—so I looked like a Teamster girl in tight jeans and a T-shirt, standing in mile-high platforms instead of hippie sandals.

Stan pulled into the parking lot right after me in his Valiant. I wondered how many decades he'd had his driver's license. Temma told me he'd dodged the draft in Canada, married and divorced, and lived underground for five years before he popped up and started running the Seattle branch of our little insurgence. That was a lot of driving.

He handed me a pile of flyers and told me to go to one end of the employees' parking lot while he took the other. The leaflets were an invitation to a meeting of rank and filers that we called "Teamsters for a Decent Contract"—just people getting together to talk about the upcoming contract and what they thought was going to go down. Not socialism, just this miserable corrupt union and shitty job. You had to start somewhere. The expiration of the Master Freight Agreement was a good place to begin—it covered every over-the-road driver in North America.

"Temma said you know how to talk to people," Stan said—apparently my only vote of confidence.

I thought, *Did she tell you that in bed?* He'd fucked half the women in the L.A. branch already. That must be where he got the advice from Temma. His latest wife was rumored to be teaching women's studies in Fresno.

What a prick he was—I'd been doing labor work in Los Angeles since ninth grade, and I bet I knew more than he did about living on the road.

Instead I was chipper. "Yeah, it'll be fine." I smiled at him like a Girl Scout. "I'm a regular 'Teamster girlfriend,' according to Sister Temma."

"*Are* you?" he said, looking at me in the face for the first time.

"Yeah, I'm sorry; what's your excuse for being here?" I said, not wanting to go where he was leading.

"Maybe I'll be a Teamster boyfriend." He flipped his wrists.

That cracked me up. It was going to be okay. Maybe he wasn't such a snob after all.

We separated. The parking lot was enormous; there must've been more than a hundred cars. No one had come out of work yet. I talked to some taco truck guys who were packing up. They liked my leaflet. I had typed, laid out, and printed this thing on the mimeo machine—it didn't look half-bad. I'd put a cartoon I liked at the top, of Teamster president Fitzsimmons and Nixon having a toast together in bed, with their feet hanging out of the sheet bottoms.

I went up to each vehicle and tucked a flyer inside the windshield wiper. I got a rhythm going with that song "Love Rollercoaster," The Ohio Players, playing in my head.

Love Rollercoaster, Child

Say What?

Why don't you ride?

Something hard punched me in the lower back, and I fell sprawling onto my hands and knees in the dirt.

"Hey girlie!"

I pushed up off my belly, my hands on fire, like the gravel had been shot into them. A squat muscular guy with worse teeth than a junkyard dog stood above me, with a wrench in his hand. He was smiling. I'd been smacked before, but neither my mother nor the nuns ever grinned at me while they were doing it.

"What's this crap you're sellin', girlie?—This is private property. You better get your can out of here."

He grabbed the goldenrod flyers in my satchel, which was still hanging from my shoulder. I scrambled to stand up, spilling most of them onto the ground. Blood was dripping on everything I was wearing, but I didn't know where it was coming from.

The wind picked the flyers up and started sailing them over the cars. I wished I could sail away with them. Already my mind was leaving the premises. I missed driver's ed for this.

My palms, that's where most of the blood was coming from, like stigmata. The pit bull-man held up his wrench again.

"Now look what you've done!" he shouted, like he was personally offended. "You little whore, you're gonna clean up this fucking lot before I stick my foot up your ass—"

We both heard a loud click, and he shut up.

It was Stan —in front of me, between me and the bad man. Instead of just his blue work shirt, Stan was wearing a work shirt with a holster. There was something in his hand, too.

He said two things. "Don't talk to the young woman like that—we're leaving now."

And to me: "Get in the car"—and threw me his keys. I caught them without a bounce.

I don't know what else he said. I ran with the keys—ran, ran, ran, like *The Gingerbread Man*—to Stan's white Valiant, climbed into the backseat, locked the doors, and threw his old-dude basketball sweats over my head. I wanted to crawl in the trunk. It was ninety degrees, but I didn't crack the window. I was freezing, shaking; my clothes were like wet rags. I'd never had a man look at me like that, like he was going to enjoy hurting me. He was a head shorter than me—even if he was twice as wide—and he'd made me pee in my pants.

"Sue!" I could hear Stan jogging up to the car. I lifted my head up to peek out the window. He didn't look hurt.

I unlocked the door and handed him his keys. He took one of my cut-up hands in his, like it was a petal. "Are you okay?" he said.

I burst into tears. Time for questions, that's when I fall apart. "Who was that?" I sobbed through my snot. "Was he from the company or the union? What did you do?"

"Hold on . . ." Stan got in the driver's seat, started up the engine, and peeled out. "I'm taking you home; this was bullshit. You never should've been here."

I cried harder. What did *that* mean? I'd failed at my assignment, because I didn't kick that bastard in the nuts? I was frozen? I was useless?—wasn't good enough to pass out a fucking flyer?

Stan pulled into the circle driveway in front of his duplex and parked at the door. "Don't move," he said.

He came around to the backseat door and opened it up, crouching down so he could look me in the eye.

"I'm sorry, I'm okay, I can get out," I said, ready for another defense. But when I glanced down at my chest, I saw my shirt was ripped open too. Who did that? I started gulping air again.

Stan put his arms around me; "Hold on to my neck," he said. He coaxed me out of the car—and once he got me to my feet he picked me up like a new bride—a bride who couldn't stop sobbing—and carried me through the front door. I don't know how he managed the lock.

He laid me down on the white sofa our other comrades had given him when he moved in two weeks ago. It had Top Ramen, pizza, and cum stains from the last ten years adding to its luster. He went to get me one of his extra work shirts to change into. I heard him take off the gun and holster. No more clicks. He came back with a bottle of povidone, the shirt, and a steaming wet towel. I had some bloody scratches on me, plus snot and sweat—not as bad as it seemed. The warm towel felt so good.

"What do you drink?" Stan said. I could hear him opening his kitchen cupboards.

"Ginger ale?"

"Yeah, right," he said and came back with two jam jar glasses and a bottle of something that said *Jack Daniel's* in flowery script on the front of the label, like an old western. "Drink up," he said, handing me the glass like it was medicine.

I took a sip. Worse than medicine! It was almost as bad as Ny-Quil. But I'd never tasted whiskey.

I gagged, and he laughed.

"Don't laugh at me; this is horrible."

"The horrible part is over—we're lucky to be alive. You're going to be okay, baby."

Baby.

"You think I shouldn't have been there," I said, "because I can't handle it, because I'm not part of the new macho Teamster campaign and I don't have a six-shooter to wave around, like I'm some freak girlfriend diaper baby."

The Jack was giving me something to talk about.

Stan said no. He said it was his fault. He said Ambrose and Ter and Aaron and Robin worshipped the ground I walked on; he said he'd been a bastard to me. Temma was right; I was sweet as pie. He tucked me in, found more blankets and a couple of pillows. I slipped on his shirt and kicked off my pants. Was he watching me?

I didn't care. I passed out on his sofa like it was the middle of the night.

I woke up with a start; I had to pee. Had it been hours or minutes? The streetlight poured in through Stan's bamboo blinds. I could see a blue clock in the corner that Ambrose had donated to our new branch organizer's furnishings. 3 A.M. It'd been twelve hours since we were in the parking lot.

Stan's apartment was two bedrooms, a living room, and a kitchen. One bedroom was the production room, with the mimeo, ditto machines, and paper supply. I crept into the bathroom next to it, the tile floor cold under my feet. Stan's shirt barely covered my ass; everything in the bathroom was icy. I thought about my warm waterbed back at my dad's house, and my fluffy cat Pooki making her nest in the middle of my quilts.

Stan appeared at the doorway.

"I'm sorry; I didn't mean to wake you up," I whispered, from the toilet.

"I'm not asleep," he said, "You say 'sorry' too much. I've been awake the whole time."

"Why?" I said, not whispering anymore. I grabbed one of his white duck hand-towels and wiped my face, getting a glimpse in the medicine cabinet mirror.

He stepped behind me and looked into my reflection. He must have been over six feet tall. Blue eyes, drooping lids. He braced his arms on the sink's edge, so I was caught in the middle between the fixture and his chest. If I moved one inch I'd be in his arms.

He spoke to me in the looking glass. "You're driving me crazy, you know that, don't you."

He said it, he didn't ask. But I still shook my head. I couldn't breathe.

"Yes, you are, the way you walk around this place, the way you smell . . ."

I could smell myself too; I could smell him, like gunpowder and Mr. Daniel's—but I couldn't speak. My legs shook a little, my knees still stinging from where the flesh had been scraped off in the parking lot. Stan felt me shiver too. He put his long hands on my shoulders and turned me around to face him so my bottom was pressed against the sink.

"You know what you're doing to me?" he repeated. He got down on his knees in one motion, parted the shirttail of the chamois I was wearing, and pressed his face right into my pussy. I grabbed the sink to stop from falling over. He steadied my thighs with his hands. His fingers were like soft sandpaper. My cunt was on his mouth, like a ball sunk into a mitt.

I'd had guys eat me out before. It'd always been an event, an antic. The Olympics of Teenage Fumbling. I wondered if they liked it or if they were just going through the motions.

But Stan wasn't like that. He was crazy; it was like he had to get inside me—he had to get his entire head in me. He was going to cannibalize me from the cunt out, put his cock in my pot and stir it until I screamed. The only way to relieve his ache was to stake me right through my cunt and take us both right down the rabbit hole. I could feel myself getting bigger and smaller every second.

"He's a great fuck . . ." Wasn't that Temma's advertisement when Stan first arrived in town? Who was she talking about? Not this man. Not where he was driving me now. This was the roller coaster no child had ever lived through. I gasped from holding my breath for so long.

Baby. Fuck me.

I couldn't speak, but he heard me. His tongue was stroking my clit and it was all I could hang on to. My legs were shaking bad and I doubled over like Raggedy Ann. Stan stood all the way up and lifted me one more time—this man was never going to let my feet touch the floor again.

I hopped onto his waist, hugging my legs and arms around him. He sank me onto his hard prick, like the last piece of a puzzle. My head dropped back. He squeezed my ass to lift me just an inch off his cock, and I whimpered. Don't make me wait.

He was going to make me.

"I'm going to make sweet belly love to your pussy 'til you come for me," he said, carrying me across the floor to his bed. His sheets were blue jersey; an *Economist* lay half-read on the floor. I bit into his shoulder, and he drove himself into me to the hilt.

Who was this man; what was this fucking? Robin, Temma— none of them looked desperate when they said his name. Their bellies didn't tremble like mine.

Baby. Susie. Come on my cock. He called my name over and over.

I'd come for him; I arched my back as if to break it. My cunt begged him. He said, "You're taking me down," like my pussy had the ammunition, but how did I ever make him turn me into his fuck doll, his mewling cat, his baby?

The head of his cock came out and teased me one more time. I cracked before he could even bury me for a final stroke. I pulled all his weight onto me, and he shuddered while I milked his cock. The tables turn, don't they. Kittens become cats. I felt ageless—he was my boy, a very big boy falling apart in my arms.

"Are you okay?" I guessed that was his big question.

Yeah, I was. I cried harder letting him pull out of me than when I'd hidden under his basketball sweats in the Valiant. Daylight was breaking. He got up to get me another whiskey and a ginger ale. I asked him if I could roll a joint, and he tossed me a Baggie from under some Emma Goldman autobiographies on the floor.

"What are you reading her for?" I asked, licking the Zigzag.

"I've been reading Emma since I was a draft dodger."

"Yeah, I heard about that. How'd you do it?"

"I wore a dress."

"Like Phil Ochs?" I threw the sheets off. "Or like a Teamster girlfriend singing the 'Draft Dodger Rag'?"

"How can you be old enough to know that song?" he said.

"I'm not."

I started it, and he caught up to me on the second line:

"Yes, I'm only eighteen, I got a ruptured spleen

"And I always carry a purse."

I reached out for him with my scabbed-up hand. "I'm not eighteen, but I know a lot of things," I said. "You underestimated me—well—I guess I thought you were an asshole, too."

"Yeah, you got that right," Stan said, and took a drag on the Thai stick. "How old *are* you?" He exhaled. "No, don't tell me."

I wouldn't. I couldn't stand to lie apart from him. I was an infant; I wanted him to cradle me and never let my toes touch the ground.

"How can I leave next week and go off to Detroit without you?—*shit!*" I said. I straddled his lap and blew a smoke ring. His blue eyes landed right in the center of my target. His cock grew hard again underneath me.

Everyone, everyone but Stan and a couple others, was heading to rural Michigan for "cadre training." This was the first moment I hadn't craved to go away. I never wanted another day to break.

"You're going to be fine," he said. "You gotta go," he said, taking the doobie from me. "There's not a man alive who's not an asshole—that's all you need to know—but you're gonna be okay." His hard-on started to soften.

Why'd he have to go and say that? Fuck, Stan.

Didn't he get it? I would tell him I loved him right then, but I knew that wasn't cool.

Instead, I moved his hand between my legs again, and the wetness shut him up. *Feel how I feel.* I leaned down to take his mouth in mine and make all the nonsense stop.

Absolutely Dangerous

Linda Gray Sexton

It was during a low, slow, hazy afternoon that I discovered a new desire in myself, and urged my lover, without words or any kind of communication, to play a brand-new game. We hadn't planned it, and neither of us had ever before experimented with erotic asphyxiation. I had read about it, and been vaguely horrified, as the practice seemed dangerous beyond reason. Why do something if you know it might kill you? I could not imagine any sexual act compelling enough that I would be willing to take the chance.

Why did the chilling statistics matter so much to me initially? One thousand people dying every year is not so many, not when compared with the figures for heart attack, breast cancer, or even car wrecks. Still, it struck me as a ghastly figure, because to die willingly, from any sort of sex, seemed suffused with depravity. Sex and death, so closely tied in some ways: the loss of self; the offering up of one's body like a sacrifice upon the temple of the bed. Why dare death?

At first other things had been enough. There had been the sex with my panties pushed aside and my butt hiked up on the bathroom's tile countertop, as we watched our rhythm in the wide three-angled mirror. There had been the night I struggled, feigning helplessness, as I let him bind me spread-eagled to the bed and use a long black dildo that we had secreted in our sex toy box the day before. There had been the day I dressed up—or didn't dress—and arrived at his house naked beneath an ankle-length black raincoat; I got spanked for that one, bent over the sofa, which was, of course, my intended purpose.

These episodes were certainly good sex, exciting sex, sex getting even better. But what about the best ever? That had to qualify in some other, magical way, complete with elusive, overwhelming qualities that weren't present in any of the other intimate encounters. Somewhere in the time that spanned the loss of my virginity to a postmenopausal woman of fifty-five, was the answer. And it didn't take me long to identify it.

As I look back, with some longing, to the episode which *does* qualify as the best, I think part of it was the element of surprise itself, the lack of the known, the idea that this was something we had never dared do before. And, perhaps most important, it was that this kind of sex was absolutely dangerous.

That day, I put his hands up and around my throat, and, seeming to intuit what I meant, he began to squeeze. The lack of oxygen made a fiery bow of my body, bent back on itself, as one orgasm after another after another rippled through me. Behind my eyelids, a rainbow of shimmering colors sucked me down into the center of my body and then out again into my fading consciousness. I was helpless before my lover and, more important, before myself. As the tatters of my self faded beneath a wild abandon, I was unable to tell him to stop. I turned myself over to him, entirely.

At this time in my career, I was working on my fourth novel, *Private Acts*. Writing fictitiously in this book was the closest I could come to admitting, via an imagined heroine, without embarrassing myself totally. I wanted to write something that spoke frankly about sex between men and women. Even so, after publication, friends would ask, "How did you find out about such sex?" And I would answer, lightly, "Imagine, imagine, imagine." I wasn't willing to take responsibility for what I had craved, or what I had done. Of course, in those days, with the exception of a few who were audacious, women writers did not often touch the topic of sex bluntly. When I used words like *fuck* and *prick* and *come*, I was scolded and even reproved for having stepped over some invisible but impenetrable barrier into inappropriate language. Those words belonged to men, and even my feminist friends criticized me for having used them.

"Gratuitous!" some said.

"As gross as men usually are!" claimed others.

"What about John Updike? Or Philip Roth?" I countered, thinking of masturbation into a piece of liver, or a woman convinced into drinking her lover's urine. What I was writing about seemed downright tame.

"You're not John Updike or Philip Roth," they pointed out. "You're a woman." I watered down my manuscript, but a few original concepts stayed with me, even though the original worksheets, in all their sweet glory, are in a cardboard box up in the attic, yellowing sheet by sheet while their words fade with age.

Yet, again and again, the editor who had bought the novel forced me to hide the true intention of my prose, even though the title of the book, *Private Acts,* most surely described the subject. I made as few of the changes as I could. All the time I was rewriting, I thought of the love I had had for this man, a man who had helped me to reveal something new about myself, to myself. Accepting him and what we had done felt imperative: I loved him without wanting to change him or our act. Could I protect that sort of love, that sort of gift, and even my detailed descriptions about what had drawn us together, while still pleasing my disgruntled editor and my horrified friends? Ultimately I did get some of what I had so wanted to include, even though it was not the way I had originally written it, because, in the end, my editor had forced me to dilute it. My heroine simply slid sideways across either side of the mattress so that the pressure of her lover's hands on the bed made an oxygenlike deprivation occur, a deprivation that made her orgasm even more intense than any other she had ever experienced.

Now, I still remember a few words and lines that had been different in the first versions of the novel. But most of the scene-altering revisions still stand in the text below. The scene still describes great sex, but it describes it in a dishonest way. In accordance with my memory, I have now changed a few things back to the way they were before my editor began to chip away at my intention like an angry sculptor: the words *cunt, prick, tongue, fuck, eats,* cut then, now are once more present. Today, I restore in parenthesis a few details and words that were the most critical to me, and which were not used. Most important, while trespassing over the editor's boundaries in the second to last line, I clarify the idea that a mattress slipping sideways cannot suffice for hands around a throat.

As is their habit, they have already been here for several hours. In this lull, they rest before returning to feast on one another. He rubs his face, slowly, back and forth in her [*cunt,*] then moves up, spreading her wetness across them both, over their bellies and thighs. Their pubic hair is matted, glistening. He enters her quickly. She comes again as he presses in to fill her, bucking her hips up in a shudder that travels throughout her body. In the last few weeks she had discovered that during a long interlude like this, it is possible for her to climax [*come*] many times, over and over, and from nothing more than a single touch or a single entry. No longer does she require a lot of time or hard work or manipulating in just the right spot. His mouth alone on her nipple or on the back of her neck or his fingers or his voice—any of it can bring her off. She looks up into his eyes and sees that the golden iris is now just a rim against the white, a sun setting into the oblivion of pleasure. He moves faster and faster until he is just a blur inside and above her, part of her. His motion casts her sideways on the mattress; her head falls over the edge, the blood rushes up [*behind her eyes*]. His chest is flushing red, his hands grasp and clutch either side of the mattress [*her throat*] on either side of her neck. [*and he squeezes*]. The window behind him throws light over his body and sets him on fire.

He pushes himself into the main artery of her body and she dances outward; blackness clouds her eyes until all she can see is his face silhouetted against the sun, rushing away from her [*as the dark increases*]; all she can feel is the pounding of his body into hers. In the fever of [*the growing blackness*], she starts to climax [*come*], again, harder than ever before: merged with him she has ceased to be herself alone. The waves break in her head and in her body and she can't *(she won't)* stop him. She would die now, all of her sex, and nothing else. She wants to go out on high, seized [*by her sex*], swept through the glass and up into the sky.

A cry, from far away, hoarse, raw. He shudders and slumps against her. His hands release the mattress [*her throat*]. She picks her head up, her lungs expand, fill with cool air, her vision clears. Her head still spins.

My urgent need to describe this kind of sex so blatantly in the novel was immense. I had discovered something important about myself—and undoubtedly about others—and I desperately wanted to write about it. I wanted to talk about it with every woman I knew; I wanted to hear that others had felt the same thing; I wanted to know I wasn't sick or strange to have experienced this kind of pleasure. I wanted to see it as an act of love and have that belief validated. And to fail to write about it in a novel so filled with sex was to fail the book and all its vital meanings.

Eventually my lover left, and I went back to more conventional sex. But I never forgot the intensity of the experience I had discovered with him on a mattress in a hot attic, stealing those few hours before my children came home from school. Over the next few years, I thought of him often, but eventually work took me from one coast to the other, and being in a new place helped me to forget those long and languorous hours spent in afternoon sex.

And then the bizarre intervened. One evening the phone rang and I heard a familiar voice on the end of the line: my old lover of so long ago had tracked me down. Now, he was moving to the exact area in which I had staked a claim for a new life. The man with whom I had experienced the best sex I'd ever had was once again within reach.

"I have incredible news," he said, with a boast in his voice. "You should probably sit down."

"I'm fine standing," I answered, figuring that he was about to tell me he had a new wife and a child in tow.

"I've had SRS."

"Which is what?"

"SRS," he answered, "is sexual reassignment surgery."

"Sexual reassignment surgery?" I repeated, still not really understanding.

"I'm not Steven anymore. I'm Stephanie."

I couldn't think of a thing to say. A vague picture flew through my mind of penises being lopped off, replaced by patchwork vaginas.

"Can't you hear it in my voice?" he asked. "Don't I sound more feminine?"

I wouldn't give him the satisfaction of saying so.

"I'm gorgeous now," he said. "I've got long black hair, beautiful breasts, legs that go on and on. I have a lot of men in my life. A lot."

Long black hair? All I could think of was how bald he had been. Beautiful breasts? All I could think of was his muscular chest. Long legs? He had only been five foot nine.

"And all my parts work just right," he said, lightly, in his now recognizably higher-pitched voice. He knew it was an indiscreet revelation, but I had the sense that he just couldn't wait to tell me that particular.

"So when can we get together?" he asked. "How about some 'girl' shopping." He giggled. "It'd be fun."

I made an excuse, hung up hurriedly, and sat on my bed, stunned. What upset me most? The fact that he was now a woman? Or the fact that though he'd once again come within reach, I'd never ever have that indescribable sex again?

Over the next year he called me repeatedly. I didn't want to see him. I was having a lot of trouble meeting men—in contrast to his brag of many partners. Mostly I spent time trolling through the online dating services, once in a while trying to find a partner, without much success. So how was he, a woman who was not really quite a woman, having so much success in the world of dating?

When I moved to another city at the end of that year, I purposely did not leave a forwarding address registered with the post office or a new phone number with PacBell, because I didn't want him to be able to find me. I didn't want to hear again that the best sex I'd ever had would probably never be repeated—at least not with that particular and willing partner. I sensed that most of the men I would eventually meet would not be interested in the kind of sex that had taken me the farthest. It was too far out on the edge, too dangerous. That, of course, was what had made it the most thrilling sex ever.

The One Who Breaks My Heart

Rosemary Daniell

You were wild once. Don't let them tame you.

–ISADORA DUNCAN

Recently, a friend suggested that I cleanse myself—as she had—of former lovers by burning a candle for everyone I'd ever slept with, and then writing prayers for them and scattering or burning the ashes. "You *must* do it!" she exhorted, her face glowing. "It's so freeing—and until you do, they're still zapping your energy, taking up room inside your head!"

"I couldn't possibly do that—there would be too many," I said, recalling the period in the late 1970s and early 1980s after my third divorce when I spread my legs and my affections, briefly, to many. What I didn't add was that I *liked* their spirits inside me—it's cozy in there, a delicious mush, and getting rid of them would feel like losing riches.

Call me a slut—and I'm sure many have—but I'm one of those women who literally can't remember all the men I've slept with (and barely all the women). And that, on reflection, should cause me to flush with shame. But it doesn't. Instead, when I do—rarely—look back on my many lovers, I'm suffused instead with a feeling of wealth—of having won the memory jackpot; like an aquarium full of exotic fish, I see them swimming, a school of beautiful creatures, flashing by so fast I can hardly catch a glimpse of any certain one.

So instead, considering myself, as actress Catherine Deneuve said, to be "too young for regrets," I stick to my credo that says it's the things we *don't do* we regret. Guilt is one of those useless emotions I refuse to indulge. Nor was I one of those women who repents, giving up freedom for the security of home and hearth. During that period between my third and fourth marriages, I got a lot of "strange," as we say in the South. And, as southern men always chivalrously add, "The worst I ever had was wonderful."

On those occasions today when I actually run into one of my former lovers—the literary community is a small town—I feel the flash of our special bond. When I hear that one or another of them has died, I experience a sudden sadness, a pang that goes deep. We shared something real—even if not "love."

In addition to sleeping with men, I've also married a lot of them. I married for the first time at sixteen, my excuse being that I had to escape my abusive, alcoholic father. At sixteen, I didn't notice that I was exchanging one raging man for another. Next came the staid-to-the-point-of-boring young architect my grandmother called "good husband material." He excelled at laying neat squares of zoysia grass in our suburban front yard. The third, an Ivy league-educated poet-cum-Boston Jewish Prince, could turn his back in bed with the best of them.

At first, during the years following my third divorce—my three kids had left home and I was living alone for the first time—the men I chose were artists, with an occasional psychologist thrown in, men I thought reflected my interests in truth and beauty, but who, I quickly learned, were also skilled at wounding me. (Once, a psychiatrist canceled our date, saying that after reading my first book, which was full of feminist rage and sexuality, he was afraid to go out with me. After our failed rendezvous, a semi-famous poet said he couldn't get it up because of my "rhetoric." I was tired of the clash of egos, the competition, among my male peers. Indeed I was discovering the truth of biographer Judith Thurman's statement about Colette, that "a man who was worthy of her would have been the road to perdition." It would have led to submission.

I left the so-called spiritually evolved men behind, and with the one goal of getting laid, began choosing from among the Others—those totally outside my class and experience. They were Too Young. They were like the decades-younger man who heard my adult daughter call me Mother and asked if that were my nickname. Or Too Dumb—like the hunky oil rigger who had seduced me on my second night aboard the oil rig where I had gone to work and clearly to get laid. Too Incomprehensible, as in the Yugoslavian ship captain with whom I learned it wasn't really necessary to be able to exchange a word of English. When I took him to a gay women's bar, he exclaimed: "Just like Yugoslavia!" Too Shady, too outside the law, like The Pirate, who conducted strange business in Belize and sometimes showed up with Hispanic bodyguards. Too Uneducated, like the swarthy younger man, exotic as a black orchid, who worked in a porn shop by day and as a male stripper at night, then sweetly cooked me meals, waiting for my approval—the one my women friends scorned, then went to see perform, stuffing dollar bills into his G-string.

The rules of seduction with these men were simple—look good, smell good—perfume, a low-necked blouse, a flower in my hair would do it—and listen, endlessly listen. It should have made my feminist heart cringe but it didn't. (Though recently, viewing *The Girl Friend Experience,* in which real-life escort and porn star Sasha Grey listens, and listens and listens to one man after another, never revealing anything about herself, I winced. I remembered myself listening to endless talk about Vietnam, Iraq, vengeful ex-wives, and ungrateful children, my eyes riveted on theirs in order meet my ends.)

After all, I wasn't looking for a relationship, I didn't have to live with them; I didn't even have to make them dinner, and being a good dancer was right up there on my list with great sex. Indeed I considered my new approach to be a form of simplification. Besides, as a writer, I could chalk it up to "research," just like the gig on the oil rig. During that period, I said I was a schoolteacher instead of a writer, not wanting to intimidate them. And even when they did find out about my rarefied occupation, they appeared unfazed. It was as though they didn't even know what a writer was—I could have said I was a peacock or from Mars—or better yet, a stripper—and they would have remained as undeterred as I was.

And believe me—some of those who were best, the most imaginative, in bed had *none* of the qualities a more sensible woman might look for in a man. But that didn't matter—in fact, the more inappropriate they were, the better. Besides retaining my personal freedom, my one goal was excitement. Without even meaning to, I had become a risk taker, a camoufleur. My erotic life was my own Mount Everest, and I wanted adventure above all.

But in the midst of these escapades, something strange happened. The delectable lifestyle I had devised for myself began to feel wearing, repetitive. Unbelievably—this was something I had never imagined—I began to feel an ennui setting in during sex with each new man.

Then, as the Goddess would have it, along came Zane.

Zane was also one of the "inappropriate" ones—a sexy, hard-drinking paratrooper fifteen years my junior. When our gaze met across a bar in 1981, I was riveted by his steel blue eyes, the Marlboro Man crinkles around them, his happy, inebriated grin. With his red-gold hair, he looked like a bronze god, or one of the muscular angels on the ceiling of the Sistine Chapel. His ragged T-shirt and cutoffs, his flip-flops, only enhanced his masculine charm, and as we talked, then danced, my hand caressing his hard, tattooed bicep, he sang "When a man loves a woman" in my ear. I quickly sized him up as a great one-night stand. When he invited me to go to his nearby apartment, where he could change in order to take me somewhere nicer, I murmured yes into his warm chest. Once there, I lay back on the waterbed, and he fell on top of me, where, with variations, he stayed until morning.

The next day, Zane visited my little Victorian flat and, wandering into my study, found the title page for my next book, *Sleeping with Soldiers,* stuck into my Hermes manual typewriter. I considered the title to be metaphorical, a play on the men I'd met—and fucked—on the oil rig. But now, it was about to be made manifest.

That night we sat on my couch, drinking Jamaican rum and talking without turning on the lights. He told me about his pending divorce, his psychotherapy, how much he loved his family in North Carolina. He had been the star football player in high school. He described his desire to join the French Foreign Legion, but he had become a paratrooper instead, and how he had wanted to go to Vietnam, only to be talked out of it by his dad—something he still regretted, and that was unimaginable to me, a war protester. A week later, he called to say he'd read my memoir, *Fatal Flowers,* the book I'd written about my southern mother's life and suicide, and my own life as an unrepentant rebel. It was a book that had scared the pants off lesser men—but not Zane. And though I still believed that whatever happened between us, I would be able to keep him at arm's length, something in my armored heart moved.

Little did I know that I'd just met a man with at least as much, if not more, determination than I had, as well as the one who would teach me just how powerless I really was.

First came his desire to live with me, whether or not I wanted a man around. We were already sleeping with each other every night, he reasoned, and within weeks, when he said he didn't want to sign another year's lease on his place, I gave in, still in the first flush of our passion.

After a few glowing months, we embarked on what would become years of drinking, fucking, and rage. Our fights, which, fueled by the booze we both drank in quantity, were like World War III and were about everything from how he could possibly be in the U.S. military to whether I had insulted all the housewives in America—e.g, his mother—by abhorring the character Valerie Perrine played in *The Border,* whether I would wear the stockings and garter belts he preferred me in, and often our fights led to bruises and broken furniture. (When I took the footboard of my maple bed in to be repaired for the second time, the carpenter was tactful enough not to ask how this had happened again.)

No longer being able to fuck around felt weird, like an infringement on my personal bill of rights. But, on the other hand, I was as jealous of him as he was of me. Later, when he was deployed to Germany for three years, my sister Anne—privy to my previous life—was amazed that I was faithful to him. She didn't know that he called me every Saturday morning at 9 A.M., undoubtedly thinking there was no way I was go-ing to talk to him with another man in the room.

Then there was our mutual desire for sensation, even sleaze. When I visited him in Europe, we delighted in an uncensored exhibition of Mapplethorpe's photographs, a live sex show in Hamburg, and visiting the red light district in Amsterdam, where he bought me a pair of red stilettos. Like me, he loved art, and we walked in awe through Käthe Kollwitz's house in Berlin, the Van Gogh Museum in Amsterdam, and the Musée D'Orsay in Paris.

And through it all we fought—on the Kurfurstendam in Berlin, on a street corner in Amsterdam, and on a boat ride up the Seine. Apparently, that night our eyes met in that bar we had seen the potential not only for great sex but also for venting the rage we had both brought into the relationship with us.

"If you ever want to marry again, you'd better do it before that book comes out," a woman friend warned me in 1984, just before

Sleeping with Soldiers, the story of my years of sexual freedom, was published. But Zane was unfazed, despite the fact that I had told the less-than-flattering truth about him and our relationship. Three years after the book came out, and six years into all this fun, like a snake coiled and ready to strike at the proper moment, he gave me the ultimatum: either marry or give up him, his beautiful body. So, despite my determination to remain free, I let him—after weeks of anxiety—put the ring on my finger. I even allowed him to lead me into a pretty little cottage no longer within walking distance of the bars where I once liked to hang out, and where I daily fought a losing battle against being domesticated. Soon I was thinking about what was in the refrigerator for dinner, looking out the window in amazement to see my sex *objet* mowing our lawn. I was losing every battle about visiting his blue-collar family in North Carolina, where the TVs in every room and the low ceilings made me realize almost to the point of nausea what I had gotten myself into.

Underlying all this—every argument, every separation—was the sex and rage to which we had both become addicted. Our relationship was like a postcard I had once read—*Having you helps me deal with the problems you bring me.* By then, I could no more think of doing without him or his passion for me, than cutting off my own hand.

Yet as all this was going on, another story was unfolding, one that, even more than our relationship, would wreak havoc on my treasured freedom: I discovered that my daughter Lily, living in New York, was addicted to heroin. A few years later I faced the fact that my son David was paranoid schizophrenic. For the next two decades—a period that will take another book to recount—not once did Zane protest my caring for them, taking them in when they needed us. A Taurus and a family animal, he became the one person in my family who supported my efforts to save them. Despite all, Zane had passed The Test, a test that was more important to me than any other.

Just when I thought I had a sex object for life—after all, he was fifteen years younger!—Zane's hard-driving life began to take its toll. In 1991, he was an infantry platoon sergeant in Desert Storm, with friendly fire deaths and suicides in his unit. Back in Germany, he began the drinking unto oblivion that would lead to the first of four rehabs, and later, to inpatient treatment for PTSD. In 1999, at age forty-eight, he had a heart attack, and then, six months later, a quadruple bypass for a triple blockage called a Widow Maker. As I sat beside his hospital bed, the love I felt for him surpassed the simple passion we had known through the years. At one point, when a staph infection invaded the site of his incision, he lay for a week with his chest open, his heart exposed, the wound cleaned and the dressings changed every six hours. I would press my cheek against his when he called out to me, and sit beside him as he endured the claustrophobia of the hyperbaric chamber he was slid into to have his infection bombarded with pure oxygen. His body and soul were mine, and I wanted to protect, enfold them.

But his near-death experience also precipitated a new round of drinking—this time, with a suicidal vengeance. For the next eight years, he drank and drank and drank—and often raged—as I lay in another room and read books and wrote. I traveled to writers' colonies and conferences, and led Zona Rosa, the series of writing-and-living groups I founded for women just before we met. When problems with my kids came up, I dealt with them alone. And sometimes, when I wasn't too furious, we had great sex despite the booze. Like most alcoholics, he was a master manipulator, good at promising me what I wanted—from tango lessons to an immediate end to all this chaos. Nor did he lose his sardonic sense of humor: When a gas heater exploded in the garage (where he'd taken to hanging out to drink and watch TV) and burned his beautiful penis, he called the scar his Aztec Surgical Modification, claiming that it added to his prowess.

Why I was faithful to him during this period, I don't know, yet I was. In truth, during those years, I frequently yearned for those times of easy, indiscriminate sex, when I didn't have to take care of anyone's feelings but my own. When Zane and I separated, as eventually happened in 2008, when he left for rehab for the last time, I had fun looking guys up on the Internet, but none of them sounded quite as interesting to me as Zane. When I saw a hunky man on the street, my next thought was almost always *but he doesn't punch my buttons like Zane.* "She liked imaginary men best of all" read a retro package of tissues that lay beside my bed with my vibrator. And while I kept thinking I would revert to my wild ways, I didn't. Also, when I did find a man attractive, it was now for different reasons—reasons that were almost protective of my relationship with Zane. These men were, inevitably, spiritually evolved, intellectual men—always married—with whom I formed deep friendships, but with whom my former behavior would have been out of the question.

Nor do I know why I didn't divorce him—after all, I'd lived through that particular scenario three times before. I was far from my grandmother, who knew she would be with the man she had married until the end of one of their lives. And then there was my shame: was I really as strong or as smart as I thought I was? And if I was, wouldn't I have left him long before? "I would have kicked him out in three weeks!" a friend said when I told her of Zane sitting for four months in what had once been my study, drinking, smoking, and watching TV with the blinds down, and occasionally saying he was going out for cigarettes, then coming back after eight hours at a bar—this, just before his last stint at a rehab and over two years spent in recovery.

The only thing I did to protect myself was to buy his half of the house from him, so that it now belongs solely to me. After all, he's the man for whom I've written the half-dozen love poems framed in my dining room, complete with my drawings of hearts, flowers, birds, ribbons. Indeed, there is homage to our love everywhere—from the photos beneath magnets on the refrigerator to the deliriously happy-looking portraits taken of us together by Bud Lee, the photographer who took the famous *Life* magazine cover of the child inadvertently hit by a policeman's bullet during the Newark, New Jersey, riots in 1967. In Savannah in the 1980s, as photos for a feature I was writing for *Mother Jones*, Bud, taken by the radiance of my and Zane's passion, had snapped the pictures.

"Sex and death are the only two things worth writing about," wrote the great poet William Butler Yeats. And when I was asked to write this essay, I was immersed in the latter. It was 2009, and my adult son, David, had just died at my home after a ten-month illness during which I had held my breath, praying every day for his healing, but also knowing it wasn't likely to happen. As I held him in my arms just after his breath expired, I placed my hands in his still-warm armpits, seeking to will him back to life, and embracing him in a way he, as an adult man, wouldn't have permitted. My most recent writing had been the memorial letter I had sent to friends everywhere.

Thus the request felt almost jarring, as though it had come from another planet. At first the idea of thinking—especially at that time—about what had been the best sex of my life seemed foreign. Then, suddenly, it seemed apropos. Hasn't my love for both of them—from the first moment I looked into my son's Cherokee-brown eyes, a dimple indenting his olive cheek as he sucked his little thumb, to the instant when Zane's steel blue eyes met mine across that bar—been undeniably of the visceral, of the flesh? "Skin," the Spanish call the first time we see one another. And hadn't I experienced the whole of my relationship with each of them in that moment?

Tonight, almost thirty years after we first laid eyes on each other, Zane and I sit at the Starbucks near my house. He, cigarette in hand, tells me that the only way he can live is not to care about anything—sex included, and even if he lives or dies. "That's evident," I say in a conversation we've had many times before: "Otherwise you wouldn't be smoking that cigarette." Once I would have argued further with him about this. But now, since we don't live together anymore, I just sit and listen.

Also, there's what we both accept as fact: to lead the simple, peaceful life he now leads—so different from his years as a paratrooper, then over-the-road trucker, outdoing himself physically every day of his life, he's had to change, giving up the rage that had fueled him for so long. He now takes Wellbutrin for depression, Depakote and lithium for bipolar, other pills for high blood pressure and for high cholesterol—sixteen each morning and eight at night. Over the past few years, he's lost his father, his mother, and his brother, so there's nobody left but me and my two daughters.

This information hangs in the air between us as we sip our lattes, talk about his latest story. Zane is writing now, too, and because he didn't come out of an MFA program, he has a lot to write about. In a few minutes, he'll leave for his AA meeting, and I mention my son, David. Because of both of them, I've seen suffering beyond what I've known myself, and I've watched their sheer male bravery in the face of it. In response, Zane quotes the Tao Te Ching—"'just stay at the center of the circle and let all things take their course.'" As he speaks, I recall reading that in the Tao, both hedonism and asceticism can lead to enlightenment, and I remember how, at one time, the former had worked for me.

And suddenly, I feel a deep peace. Can it be that this man—the one who once drove me mad with his stubbornness, his need to dominate—the one I once considered the almost unmovable obstacle to my personal freedom—has become my unlikely spiritual guide?

Also, there is our separation of over two years, which has led us to see each other with new eyes. "Don't think I take any of this for granted," he said the other night as we cooked dinner together in my kitchen. And yes, while our earlier relationship had been rife with passion, the price had been a rage that would have put Elizabeth Taylor and Richard Burton to shame. But the ardor that moves us now is no longer fueled by fury. As Eckhart Tolle writes, when we observe and let go of the pain body—all that we previously blamed on the people around us—we are free to either separate with love or to enjoy an ever-deepening relationship.

As I run my fingertips over the now-even-deeper grooves beside his eyes, I sense that something delightful is about to happen—that my sensual life is about to begin again. Once again everything is open-ended—I don't quite know what will happen next—and along with the moments of anxiety that causes, I like it that way. So am I—as I'm now free to do—about to pull a Jane Juska, go wild once more, reverting to my old ways? Or am I simply about to share something new with this stranger I've known for so long?

And whether what is to come will be with Zane, or with some other man (or even woman), I know that it will be different. Zane, along with my kids, has taught me suffering, and suffering has changed me. His healing and Lily's, along with David's death and our closeness to my older daughter, Christine, has made us a family. What I want now is to be moved, as I was recently by the psychotherapist in my writing workshop in Santa Fe who was in tears as he read his piece about having to tell his wife she had cancer.

As I think about these things, Zane gives me that lazy grin I love so much—being bipolar has its perks, just as in our first, tempestuous years, when he would wake beside me, smiling and pulling me close, no matter how bad our fight the night before—and places my hand beneath the table and on the crotch of his jeans. And I think of the times we've had in bed lately—as seamless, as smooth and delicious as melting French chocolate.

Yes, at this moment, Zane is still the one who breaks my heart. Can it be that, at last free of doubt, I'm about to have—the best sex I've ever had?

Do I Own You Now?

Daphne Merkin

Girls in their summer dresses we know about, but what about boys in their summer bathing trunks? Him, in particular, his long-legged body, not hideously six-packed in the current style, but elegantly constructed—beautiful even, in an antelope kind of way. His smooth olive-toned skin tanned to an almost non-Caucasian pitch, and my own much lighter skin burnished to a red-brown by incessant and patient exposure.

He always wore the plainest of business suits, black or navy, not a man to take sartorial chances—or risks of any sort, really, except in bed, where he kept leading me forward, closer to the precipice, that moment where you drop off the boundary of your own precarious identity and into someone else's terrain. *Do I own you now?* he used to ask me breathlessly after some particularly entwined bout of lovemaking. Neither of us tended to speak much during sex, except for his habit of punctuating the silence with cursory yet infinitely flattering statements like *Someone should bottle you* after he rose up from below. So the ownership question came out with the force of a mission statement, one I signed off on. That summer, at least, he owned me. What was the point in pretending otherwise?

Who can forget a summer swimming in sex? Even now, far from those days and that sort of abandon, I have only to conjure up that time, more than two decades ago, to feel cramped with longing, a sensation of something dropping deep inside of me. That was also the summer I was introduced to a kind of sex I hadn't yet let myself in for, either because I wasn't available or it wasn't. Nothing to do with nipple clamps or threesomes or licking honey off a prone and naked body—none of that would have appealed to me then, as it doesn't now. No, it had to do with the way he took forever about gliding himself into me and the way he propelled me into new positions, and new submissions as well, not overtly of the S-and-M kind, but with a subtext that always hovered around the issue of power, intimating at the unspoken questions: *How much do you want this?* And, *What are you willing to do for it?*

I can still recall, as though it happened the day before yesterday, walking out of the ocean that Saturday, aware of him studiously pretending not to watch me from where he lay on his towel. I was pleasantly conscious of the way the brief dip had made my already conspicuous nipples stand out and the way my wet, slicked-back hair brought out the angles of my face. That was the summer my body was quite something in a black one-piece. I've always preferred the subtle eroticism of one-pieces to the soft porn of bikinis, but sometimes I wonder if these were the kind of nuanced distinctions that drew us apart in the first place. That, and his wish to torture me, not in a good, tantalizing way—although he did that well too—but in a steely withholding style that made me madly in need of sustenance, like a hungry baby nuzzling for a nipple.

For a while, I was willing to do anything. Bend over with my head on the bed and my ass high in the air so that he could stick his finger way up in there and then enter me from underneath, like a ship coming into its berth, filling me out perfectly. I liked that part of my body paid attention to, warmed in preparation for what would come next. I also liked neither of us seeing the other's face, which position is often taken to be intrinsically dehumanizing, but which I found to be the best way of freeing myself from the endlessly scrutinizing aspect of sex. For a while after we parted (the final time we parted, I should say, since by then parting itself had become a kind of coming together), I would lie on my bed and try to reenact this particular position in my mind—a monologue pretending to be a dialogue, bent over on my bed and envisioning him entering me from behind.

He took up all the available space in my head that summer, even though I was supposed to be busy pursuing my Higher Literary Calling. To which end I had gone off at the beginning of July to spend a month at Yaddo, a writers' colony in Saratoga Springs, New York. You had to jump through various hoops in order to be accepted to the place—fill out an application, gather recommendations, and send off samples of your writing. I guess I should have been flattered that they took me, someone with only a sheaf of book reviews and two published short stories under her belt, but what hope did Yaddo, with its mosquitoes, its self-conscious poets and networking novelists, have of holding me when he (for want of anything else, I'll resort to the slightly French affectation of using initials and call him J.C.) was back in New York City? I wanted his hands on my breasts and then sliding down my body, as though he were just discovering my contours all over again. I wanted him inside me, or lying, exhausted by exertion, next to me as we slept.

For ten days, I went dutifully to my studio in the woods and tried to write. I think in all that time I managed to finish only the second half of a book review I had started back in the city, when I wasn't lying by the pool or talking with other Yaddo residents at dinner about suitably bookish things. Mostly, I was lost in visions of J.C. playing with his yellow rubber duck in the bath, J.C. tracing and retracing his long fingers around first one of my nipples and then the other, J.C. putting his mouth on mine as if he were planning to suck the air out of me, kissing me with consuming but unslobby ardor. What was it about the tip of his penis that so moved me when he began to put it between my legs, that soft velvety tip? This seemed far more important for me to parse out than why—for the sole purpose of improving my own standing in the colony's tacit but very obvious hierarchy of talent—Walker Percy's *The Moviegoer* was my favorite contemporary novel, or why X was so inexplicably over-rated as a critic when Y's was so clearly the better mind.

On the second Friday at Yaddo, I gave up on the charade. I first booked a round-trip train ticket, so as not to lose my blinding sense of intention, and then explained to the writer who ran the colony with his much older (and more famous) wife that a dire family emergency had suddenly burst over the horizon and required my immediate but short-lived attendance back home. I was torn, I assured the director, about whether to go and interrupt this extraordinary opportunity to convene with the woods *à la* Thoreau, but I would make it as quick a stay as I could. He bought into my bald excuses with utmost grace. How was he to know that under my serious-seeming writerly self was a creature deranged by sexual longing, an updated and less provincial version of Madame Bovary, dying to escape her small-town existence and have another fling with the callous Rodolphe?

I was back in the city and in J.C.'s low and not particularly comfortable bed by Friday evening, but something had gone wrong by the next day, after we had subwayed and ferried over to Fire Island. I may have said something mocking but affectionate that he took to be merely mocking; he was always misreading my tone that way. I only know that by the time I walked out of the ocean, we were no longer on speaking terms. J.C. ignored me as I settled myself back on the expansive beach towel he had brought; he continued to lie silently on his side of the towel, his arms folded behind his head and his eyes closed as he gave himself up to the peak rays. I lay on my stomach, staring out onto the crowded beach that seemed to shimmer in the heat, wondering why I had ever succumbed to a man who, right from the start, disliked me as much as he lusted after me. For the next hour or two, as the afternoon grew cooler and my skin took on the crunchy texture of sand mixed with tanning cream, we continued to coexist without a word passing between us. I made several firm decisions in my head, scrambling to find a foothold in the chaos of J.C.'s intermittent affections. (1) I would pay more attention to my writing when I returned to Yaddo. (2) From here on in, I'd stop trying to endear myself to men who viewed me with a mixture of hostility and curiosity, as though I were an exotic species of female that happened to crawl out from under a rock. (3) On a more specific level, I would try to bring this day to a close without getting teary or angry, and then, calling on whatever lingering strength of character I had, I would put J.C. and his bedroom skills behind me forever.

Somewhere between leaving the beach and the ferry ride, we started talking again. Once he decided he had been punitive or distancing enough, J.C.'s relational style was to act as if nothing had ever gone awry—no rift, no icy walls put up between us. By this point, I was so reduced by his ability to leave me behind like a piece of debris that I embraced the chance to be part of a couple again, my girlfriend to his boyfriend. It was in this humbled but also agitated spirit that I went back to his apartment with him. He warmed up some uninspired leftovers, and we sat at the small half-circle of a table that stood against an unwelcoming bare wall in his minimalist studio apartment and made desultory conversation. I had spent 10 days at Yaddo daydreaming about going to bed with him, which was why I went home with him rather than holding my head up high and bidding him a collected adieu the minute we hit the city. I assume he knew this as well as—if not better than—I did, but at some point I gathered up the few remaining shreds of false dignity I had and murmured that I had to make the last train back to Saratoga Springs. As if on cue, J.C. got up and sauntered over to his bed, which was all of a few feet away, and lay down on it. *Come over here,* he said. *You don't really want to go now, do you? I bet I know what you want.*

You bet he did. What's the point of fighting the insinuating nature of desire when it won't leave you alone, won't shut up until you attend to it? I walked over to the far side of J.C.'s bed and stood there shyly, like a girl fresh off a Nebraska farm. I was wearing a long, flimsy summer skirt, and I stood there silently, wondering how to move the scene forward without completely selling myself out. And then, in his deft, wordless way, J.C. rolled toward my side and pulled me toward him. He stared into my face with his large, somewhat wary brown eyes, as though he understood that things were difficult for me, a girl dealing with too many inner conflicts (none of which, it was understood, had anything to do with him), and then he put his hand up under my skirt and pulled down my underpants—not all the way down, but somewhere in the vicinity of my ankles. He continued to watch me closely as he put his hand up under my skirt.

The frenzied feeling of being away from him, followed by the thwarted day at the beach, followed now by the way he seemed to coax me into my own need for him, all worked in desire's favor. You feel so milky, he said, as he continued to keep his finger inside me. When he came inside me, smelling of Old Spice and the faintest whiff of something musky coming off his skin—he was the most excretion-less man I've ever been with, I don't think I ever saw him sweat—it all made sense again. *Do I own you now?* he asked, as though the whole point of our tortuous dance was to corral me like some undomesticated beast and lead me on a rope into the tent he had pitched against the encroaching darkness. *Yes,* I whispered, like I always did.

I returned to Yaddo the following day, after J.C. went to work, dressed in his aspiring professional uniform, but by then it was already too late to pretend I was serious about becoming part of a writerly community. I was a loner at heart, looking to be taken up by another loner—someone who understood that under my barricaded demeanor I was bursting to open my gates to the next proprietary male. Ownership made sense to me, it always had, suggesting a kind of safety in confinement. It couldn't last, of course, that kind of is-this-love-or-is-this-hate entanglement, but I swear it makes my brain smoke just to consider it all these years later.

Let's Not Talk About Sex

Julie Klam

Do you want to hear something embarrassing? My daughter who is just turning six thought until last week that her vagina was called "the front." And I told her the right word because she asked why boys have penises and girls just have fronts. If I could've gotten away with never naming a body part other than the tushy, I would've. The reason she knew the word *penis* is because we have one boy dog and three girls. One day she said, "Mom, what is that?"

And I took a deep breath and said, "A penis." Because, you know, I'm very forward thinking and progressive. I just said *penis* right like that for the first time in her six years.

And she looked at me and said, "Do all boys have them?"

"Yes," I openly confirmed, "they do."

"Are they really sad that they have them?" she asked, genuinely concerned.

"No, darling," I broke it to her. "They're quite pleased with them."

Thus ended the sex talk.

I know I'm warped. I had to write about sex once before, and my face was red for a month. I actually gave myself rosacea. The piece was about making your man better in bed—ick, I wanted to scream at "your man" and "better in bed." (I still think "better in bed" means more hours of sleep.) I wrote from the point of view of the Victorian school marm I see myself as. A little more modest than Sister Wendy. It was like a challenge from the universe (in the form of a glossy women's magazine). Write about the stuff that makes you want to cringe and curl up like a roly-poly bug. I was paid the most money I'd ever made, not only that, after I wrote it, dozens of foreign magazines optioned it for years after, and I kept getting paid again. Clearly this was a topic other people had less trouble with than I.

I am not the product of an all-girls Catholic school upbringing. Oh no, I grew up in a very open, liberal, hippy-ish household. Nary a day went by when I didn't have to see someone's tushy. My parents were fiercely naked. When I got to the age where I finally demanded that my dad cover up around me, I still had run-ins with him because he was always being naked somewhere. Rather than walk inside and use the bathroom, he goes behind a tree. My mother's a nudie, too. My husband has said he's seen my mother naked (accidentally) more than he's seen me. They love being without clothes! They have an outdoor shower with nothing to keep someone from seeing you naked, except an alert system—a thumbtacked playing card by the back door that leads to the shower. A queen if a girl is taking a shower and a king if it's a male. If someone happens to be walking around the back of the house though, then they won't know about the playing card. My parents sleep naked; they swim naked. Whereas if I could shower wearing a T-shirt and underwear, I would. And before you wonder, I did once hear them doing it. I wanted to pour boiling oil in my ears. If evil governments are really looking to torture prisoners, they should forget waterboarding and just make them sit in a room beside their parents having loud sex. I'd talk!

When I was in the eighth grade trying to grow up normally in the bucolic town of Katonah, New York, one of my high school-aged brothers was regularly having sex with his girlfriend—in his bedroom—down the hall from me. I came home from school one day, and he and his girlfriend were coming out of the shower together, she a giggling mass of boobies and bubbles. I went down the hall to my pink room, closed the door, and sat on my bed with my hands folded and decided I would make it my business to find a good Jewish convent.

Very reluctantly, I went on a date with an actual boy, my first, shortly after that. Here's how it went. Cliff Covey, a ninth grade Lacrosse stud, asked his guy friend to ask his girlfriend if she would ask me if I'd go to the movies with him. I passed the note back and said yes. A lot of girls liked him; I was not one of them. Still, the idea of having contact with a boy, with your friend and her boyfriend acting as go-between, seemed like something I could handle.

I was told by my friend, the operative, to meet him at the movies. Everyone in school went to the same movie theater on Friday nights and whatever was playing was what you saw, whether it was *Pippi Longstocking* or *Das Boot*. That night it happened to be Peter Sellers in *Being There*. A perfect junior high date movie.

During the day I felt nervous, not like a happy giddy anxiety, more like a gallows walk feeling. I thought a lot about what to wear. I still considered dressing up in terms of my Jewish high holiday outfits. I had a pastel flowered skirt that had a matching French-cut T-shirt with a pocket in the same pastel flowered pattern that I wore with a lavender string and ceramic necklace and white sandals. I sat in the backseat of my mother's car after school while she and my Aunt Mattie, who was up visiting us from Manhattan, ran errands to The Mousetrap, our town's cheese shop and the Village Market, where Mattie looked into the butcher's eyes and said, "This is the most gawjus meat I have evah seen!" My mother told Mattie I was going on my first date. "Mazel tov!" she said, tapping her cigarette ashes out the window. "Don't let him feel you up." She and my mother laughed; I didn't know what that meant.

I came home and got dressed and my brother told me the outfit was stupid. I should wear jeans and "like a cool shirt." I was totally clueless. I had another skirt outfit with strawberries on the skirt and the shirt. I had no idea that dressing for a date was different from dressing to go out to dinner with my grandparents.

My mom drove me to the movies, and I felt ill the entire way. How did I get myself into this? I would've rather been home watching *Family Ties* with some blueberry cake and ice cream. We got there and I wordlessly got out of the car, silently cursing my mother for borning me into the second sex. The movie had already started; everyone was inside. I opened my pink Perry Ellis purse and pulled out my money and bought my ticket, looking at the kid in the booth with deep envy. Through the darkened theater, my eyes adjusting, my feet sticking to the floor, I found the one person who wasn't coupled up and making out: my date. He'd saved me a seat. I don't remember if he said hello before he put his arm around me and then proceeded to paint my throat with his tongue. You know a kiss is top-notch when after it ends you have need of a tennis towel to wipe your face. Each kiss was punctuated with me turning away and blotting my face into my sleeve. Blech! This went on for an hour or so, at which time Cliff asked me if I would "go out with him," i.e., go steady.

I looked at the screen. *What was Peter Sellers doing? Was he retarded? What was this movie? Where were the grown-ups?*

"Sure," I said gamely, even though I felt like I was serving a sentence. The very idea of saying no or even I don't know didn't occur to me. I'd read *Forever* by Judy Blume, and I could safely say I felt no tingling anywhere except where I'd missed some of his saliva on my cheek.

"Are you going to our lacrosse game tomorrow?" he whispered.

"Yes," I said robotically.

"It's an away game," he said. "How will you get there?"

I sat in silence and shrugged, watching Chauncey Gardner falling from one situation to another, not unlike me and this giant tongue in the Lacoste shirt. When the movie ended we said good-bye and went out of the theater, and I race-walked to my mother's station wagon in the sea of other parents' cars.

I got in and slammed the door.

"How was it?" she asked.

"Okay," I said morosely and looked out the window. My mother squeezed my leg.

When I got home my two brothers were giddily waiting at the top of the staircase to taunt me for being in luh-huh-huh-huh-hove. I walked up the stairs with grim determination like I'd just come home from taking the bar exam.

"Julie," my brothers sang, "did you enjoy your night of passion?" they said in Robin Leachy voices, gleefully taunting me until they noticed I wasn't smiling.

"What happened?" one said.

"It was horrible," I murmured. "I hated it." I went on to tell them about the Saint Bernard-style make-out session I'd endured from this ninth grade spittoon. They were almost angry with me.

"That's what you have to do!" one said.

"You better get used to it!" the other added.

They left me in my room. Was it true? Did I have to get used to that? Was this the thing that everyone else in the world actually *enjoyed*? How could I have possibly gotten it so wrong? How would I be able to keep it up? My face was already covered in a mild diaper rash. I lay awake all night, thinking about my friends joyously sneaking out of their houses to kiss boys. Something was really off with me, but I didn't care what my brothers said. I wasn't ever going to get used to it.

On Monday morning, I went to Cliff Covey's locker and broke up with him. I actually said, "I really don't think this is working out."

After that, I stuck to crushes on movie stars and staying home with my friend Barbara, who also didn't date, on Friday nights. We'd watch movies and plot how when we grew up we'd marry Kevin Bacon and Matthew Broderick. It was safe . . . and they seemed dry.

It wasn't until college that I started kissing again. The first guy I kissed was a fellow film major. He was nothing special, just kind of funny and dorky, and we all went to see *The Manchurian Candidate* together. He sat next to me and sort of let his leg hit my leg. After, he walked me home and kissed me. It was nothing like I'd remembered. Soft and slow and sexy and at no time did he test my gag reflex. I was still really scared of boys, and so when he asked me out again I made up a story about some far-off boyfriend in England whom I'd broken up with but now we were getting back together.

Now it wasn't the kissing, that was fine. But there was something terrifying in that all of the moves came from the boys. So after we kissed, then what? Would I have to take my shirt off? Or my pants? I had sat in that Peter Sellers movie like a dumb robot saying yes to everything and then my brothers told me that was how it was supposed to be. I just didn't want anything to do with it. In my brain, I thought being with a man meant giving over any personal choices and becoming a Stepford gal. A good kiss would lead to being felt up and then sex and moving in and no longer being able to choose my own TV shows or restaurants to order from. That just sounded terrible. So I abstained, oh, not out of choice, I made myself believe. Just suddenly, no one was interested in me and I decided it was because of those ten pounds I had to lose . . . and my nails were a mess . . . and my bangs hadn't grown out. I also equated the idea of having sex with letting go, being loose and out of control and unbuttoned— kind of like my yicky naked parents. That brought me back to my eighth grade self, who hadn't been able to say no or slow down.

Did I get "better"? Sure. Never underestimate the power of twenty-six years of therapy. I needed to stop seeing myself in relation to my parents and my brothers to become comfortable with who I am. And one day, I'm going to educate my daughter about sex. She's already started asking me about it. Fortunately, I stammer so long she loses interest. But soon enough, it's going to come, that moment. . . .

Violet: Mommy, where do babies come from?

Me: Why don't you ever ask me where hot dogs or Barbies come from?

Violet: Please tell me.

Me: (Sigh) Oh fine. How would you like a box of raisins?

(She stares at me.)

Me: Okay, this is hard for me to talk about because I'm not comfortable with the topic, but I certainly appreciate your need to know. (And here's where I will start double-talking her with psychological shit about repression and then maybe cough and cough and I'll ask for a glass of water and then hopefully, God willing, my bursitis will flare up.) And if none of that works, and my back's against the wall, I will pull two chairs beside each other and together we will Google it.

My Best Friend's Boyfriend

Fay Weldon

On the occasion that I lost my virginity, I was, I remember, wearing a dreary sage green woollen dressing gown. It had been run up on the sewing machine by my mother in the interest of my warmth and decency. Glamour did not come into my mother's vocabulary, though words like *prudence* and *dignity* did.

When my boyfriend—though actually he was my best friend's boyfriend, and an ex-serviceman—saw the dressing gown, he laughed, I had no idea why.

I was eighteen. It was a long time ago, in 1949 to be exact. Already you will be working out my age, so I will spare you the bother and explain to you that I am seventy-nine. Between forty-five and seventy it is only sensible for a lady writer to disguise her age, try not to let slip that she was around at the time of the Korean War, the original *Invasion of the Body Snatchers,* the invention of the pill, Watergate, and so on—but after seventy-five some other element enters in: you are so old you gain shamus status and people tend to hang on your words, no matter how foolish they may be, impressed because you still have the capacity to say them. Just get through the forty-five-to-seventy-five bit and you'll be fine.

For most women these days, I daresay, their first sexual encounter is not going to be much to write home about, let alone text or Twitter: it will have been a gradual escalation from one intimacy to another. But in 1949, sex was a private and secret activity, and not the focused rush to orgasm by all possible means that it is today. Anything but the missionary position was considered indecent and unnecessary—and some indeed were actually illegal—and no nice girl supposed it to be anything else. Rather, it was about the creation of new life, and the problem was to have the sex but not have a baby. Contraception was up to the male and consisted of "I'll only put it in a little way" or "I'll withdraw, I promise." Which was pretty much the same as no contraception at all. As a result sex was a dangerous thing, far more interesting and erotic than it is now. This; this summonsing to the bed (or in my case the floor of the student pad) of the forces that create new life, mixed up and heady with a sense of the forbidden, a fear of pregnancy, and an understanding that what you are doing was a deliberate act of social outrage, made the event remarkable.

And besides, I had been fed, on the rug, before the fire, almost a whole half bottle of Cointreau, a sticky sweet orange liqueur, which I still choose today if circumstances arise, rather than brandy or grappa or whiskey, in order to feel a whisper of that same breathless excitement, that mixture of lust, languor, fear, and sin. If the women of Catholic countries today still choose to obey the decree of the pope in Rome and avoid contraception, it isn't that they're out of their minds; it's that they just like the sensations of significant sex.

It was more curiosity than love, I admit, which drove me on. The one who plied the Cointreau was my best friend's boyfriend, she being out of town for the night. After that, I fell in love with him quite desperately, and he would climb the stairs to visit me whenever she went away, which was never often enough, and many was the night I spent secretly weeping and mad with jealousy. She was quite conceited and viewed me, I think, as plain, fat, and funny (which I was at the time) and didn't see me as any kind of danger. I showed her!

Men were rare and exotic creatures. I lived until I was fifteen in New Zealand, in an all-female household composed of my mother, my grandmother, and my sister. I went to an all-girls school. Nor was my mother keen on male company—my father was a charming philanderer and my mother virtuous, but he divorced her when I was five on the grounds of a single night's infidelity on her part, and the injustice rankled. She did not marry again. "What me, wash some man's socks?" Her reluctance mystified me. To sleep in the same bed as a man seemed to me the highest good and still does. (I was paid half a crown a page to learn John Stuart Mill's *Subjugation of Women* by heart, and concepts of highest good and so forth came easily to me.) It must be so warm and companionable under the blankets. But Mother was having none of it.

Not just rare and exotic, men were liable to turn on the instant into wild and unrestrained beasts. "Always be careful not to lead a man on: if you do they can't stop themselves," we nice girls were told. But stop what? We had only a vague idea. It is hard for younger generations to realize the extent of our ignorance on sexual matters. No girls of my acquaintance had ever seen a naked man, very few men a naked girl. Parents did not appear unclothed in front of children. Only in the *National Geographic* magazine did you get a glimpse of dusky female breasts. No TV, no computers, no Internet porn. What men and women did together was a mystery, and you didn't let your mind go there.

When we moved to England in 1946 I hoped things might be different, but no . . . I was fifteen. Still no men. Another all-girls school. No dating (a newfangled concept anyway) until you were out of school uniform. More warnings. "It's bad for men's health if they're stopped. They get pains. You must be considerate." So in consideration for male health, as we grew into women, we wore blouses buttoned up to the neck and sleeves buttoned at the wrist, lisle stockings with suspender belts to keep them up (their erotic possibilities unexplored), and an elastic girdle over the hips to make sure the shape of the body didn't bring itself to male attention. And we kept our eyes discreetly lowered in case somehow by mistake we "led men on." A friend's brother kissed me when I was sixteen and said I had nice thighs, but that was the sum of my sexual experience.

On my eighteenth birthday I arrived at the University of St. Andrews in distant Scotland, lured by the pull of the scarlet gown the students wore then and still do today, with my one suitcase of decent clothing plus the green cloth dressing gown my mother had made for me. It was so bulky the suitcase would barely shut. On that same day she closed up our home, her maternal duty done, and went to live as a bohemian in St. Ives, in even more distant Cornwall. She'd whirled the map and put in a pin and that was where it landed. That was how, in our house, decisions were made. And I was on my own, without a home, without a country, and only a scholarship from a benign state for company.

But here at the last were all the men, a 20 percent female-to-male quota (girls were seen as so *dangerous* to male morality), and a high proportion of the men were back from the wars on ex-servicemen grants. They were grown men in their twenties, and we girls were straight out of school. I hated my own ignorance. It was my instant ambition to lose my virginity. This turned out to be oddly difficult, partly I suspect because of my total lack of feminine wiles, and partly because men were not all lascivious, predatory beasts, but decent, and knew that sex led to babies, and babies led to marriage.

Virginity is a vague kind of concept these days, there being so many stages between childhood and the breaking of a hymen that many would be at a loss to remember or describe when it ceased to be. But then, moving on into the 1950s, virginity was a kind of concrete, before-and-after reality; a thing you "lost" at your peril, because a woman was obliged to live on the goodwill of men—being rarely able to earn enough to support herself. So you remembered all right. And reputation was important. You certainly did not want the name of the village bicycle, the one everyone rode.

But I was bold. I moved out of the hall of residence and rented a house with three other free-thinking girls. Hall was all rules. You were allowed men visitors in your room at teatime, but you had to move your bed out into the corridor first. It was embarrassing.

And it was one evening when the house was empty that X—I cannot bear to give you his name: I don't know quite why, but it feels like a disloyalty—pulled up on his motorbike—ah, the thrum, thrum, thrum, all that—and found me there alone, sitting on the floor beside the fire with my books, and sat beside me, and we opened my best friend's bottle of Cointreau. He didn't even have to ring the bell because in those days no one felt the need to lock front doors. He'd just come in. And before long he said "supposing you go and put on something more comfortable," and puzzled but obedient I went upstairs and came down in my sage green wool dressing gown, which was the only thing I could think of, and he laughed. But laid on top of the rug it was thick enough to make the floor really quite comfortable, or at any rate not sufficiently uncomfortable to worry, and my bed too far away to get to anyway, and I realized, my eyes finally unlowered, that he was beautiful, with glossy black hair and full red lips and a skin so different from my own, raspy where mine was silky. And even as I was coming to terms with the remarkable way my female body suddenly linked together with the male in the fashion evolution had clearly designed them for—I once watched a shapeless tadpole take its first breath on dry land: and it turned before my eyes into a baby frog, exquisite and articulated and full of bright awareness—how do we *know* how to do all this— I was born again: I turned from girl to woman. Actual sensation beyond this I cannot remember, if only because I was in the far corner of the ceiling, looking down with fascination at what was going on between the man and the girl: an out-of-body experience, but it scarcely mattered.

A psychoanalyst told me later the out-of-body experience was a symptom of shock, but I don't think so—I was just becoming part of something greater than me, whose servant I was to be. And even since then I have been convinced not just of the significance and marvel of sex, but also of its sanctity, and its healing power, and the importance it plays in our lives, and how it is wrong to deny this. And if for a time thereafter, as I fled from bed to bed in search of love, I became a positive priestess of Aphrodite, it was not for long. I had a baby, as I was bound to, and steadied up. The psychoanalyst told me I suffered from low self-esteem, but my version is I was just born to like sex, and inherited the tendency from my father.

The Diddler

J. A. K. Andres

It's an idyllic, cloudless afternoon when Callie's kindergarten teacher blindsides me. She points at my daughter, hard at work at a pint-size desk. Callie's so focused on tracing a map of Australia she hasn't noticed I've arrived.

"She's been doing that all day," her teacher says.

"Doing what?"

"The squirming," she whispers.

Callie's perched on the very corner of her seat, wriggling away. *Oh, shit,* I think.

I've seen plenty of diddlers. Little boys' hands wander down their shorts at restaurants, little girls rub against the fire pole on the playground. Their mothers yank them back to reality with a hiss: "Don't *do* that!"

I've been lucky. My older children, both boys, weren't diddlers. Now my third, my only daughter, might be having a personal relationship with a chair.

On the walk home we stop at a park and the baby crawls on the grass while Callie swings on the monkey bars. She doesn't seem interested in the fire pole.

Then she reaches under her skirt and squeezes her Hello Kitty undies.

"Callie, why are you doing that?"

"This?" She grabs her undies again. "It feels funny."

I hope she means funny as in itchy, not funny as in tingly. Then guilt rushes through me. Do I really wish my daughter were rashy rather than diddly?

"Well, just don't do that in public. Please."

At home, after I nurse the baby and switch up the laundry and marinate some chicken for dinner, I tell Callie I have to check her vagina. "I just need to see what it looks like."

"Oh, Mom," says Callie, a hint of disdain in her voice. "I already know what it looks like."

"You do?"

"It looks like boneless chicken breast."

So much for Georgia O'Keeffe's orchids.

And while I do convince Callie to show me her vagina, if I get too close she bursts out giggling.

"That tickles!" she gasps, slamming her thighs shut.

Callie's labia looks irritated. Perhaps it was red before she got friendly with her chair. I grab some diaper rash cream from the baby's room.

Writhing hysteria ensues. "Mom! Stop!" She's laughing so hard she's practically crying. I suggest Callie apply the ointment herself and leave her alone.

There's laundry to fold, the baby won't go down for a nap, my mother-in-law calls. The boys get home from school and require lumberjack-size snacks. An hour's gone by since I left Callie in her room with the ointment.

I peek in. Callie's bare-assed, in a full straddle, bent over her vagina with a limberness Nadia Comaneci would envy.

"Callie?"

"Mom! Look! You gotta see this!"

I step around her outstretched toes. She's got her clitoris in her fingertips and is giving it a twirl.

"Oh, my," is all I can say.

"Isn't this cool? It feels great! You should try it!"

At breakfast the next morning, Callie announces her vagina has a name.

"It's called Cho Cho."

One of her brothers spews milk all over his toast. The other is politely interested.

"Cho Cho? That's a weird name. Our first baseman calls his wiener Big Frank."

The baby just gurgles, a noise not unlike the one my husband makes in his throat as he glares at me over his coffee.

Days later, in a rare moment alone with my husband, I attempt to work out how Callie went from detachedly describing her vagina in meat counter terms to naming it, like a pet.

"Newtonian elation," I conclude. Finding her clitoris is to Callie what discovering gravity must have felt like to Isaac Newton.

He sighs. "Is she young for this? I mean, when did you start?"

I try to remember when I realized my vagina had a purpose beyond excretion, but no "Aha!" moment comes to mind. It was there, it was nice, but it didn't rate a nickname. These days I think of my vagina as the place my four kids came from, just as my breasts are udders dressed up in a brassiere.

Somewhere between that forgotten moment of discovery and my evolution into a vessel of motherhood, I progressed from "hurry up before my roommate comes back" dorm sex to first-apartment all-nighters to indulgent B&B weekends. Now it's solely marital-bed sex, which is a lot like hurry-up dorm sex on high-thread-count sheets. Did all that emanate from kindergarten diddling?

My husband grows bored with my slack-jawed lack of response. "Forget I asked. How do we get her to stop?"

"Stop?" That hadn't occurred to me. "I told her it's OK to play with her Cho Cho—in private. Not in front of other people, not even me."

"And not in school!"

"Of course! But, honey, I don't want her getting a hang-up about it. It's not *bad*."

"I know it's not bad," he says. "But is it normal?"

"In theory." But this isn't theory. It's our six-year-old daughter.

He turns to the computer.

"Are you Googling it?" I ask. "When girls start masturbating?"

"No," he says. "I'm going to craigslist. To search for a chastity belt."

Soon, Callie's Cho Cho is part of the family.

In the tub: "Callie, wash behind your ears, under your arms, and don't forget your Cho Cho."

At bedtime: "I wanna go commando tonight, Mom. Cho Cho needs to air out."

Watching me change the baby's diaper: "Poor baby has a wiener, not a Cho."

One afternoon, the boys yell through the house, "Hey, Mom! Make Callie put some clothes on! Our friends are coming over and we don't want them seeing her Cho Cho!"

I yell back, a bit too shrill, "Callie! Put your Cho Cho away! Now!"

She's dressed before the friends arrive, to my relief. But I also feel something akin to grief. Is this the beginning of the end of Callie's innocence?

Callie's always run around naked and carefree like a wood nymph. At six, she's in love with herself in a way she never will be again. She doesn't have long before she starts comparing herself to other girls, before she wants to wear a bra instead of nothing at all. I'd like her to stay naked and carefree as long as possible.

But when our house is teeming with eight- and ten-year-old boys, Callie the Wood Nymph seems more like Callie the Exhibitionist. It's unfair to restrain her youthful exuberance so her brother's friends don't get an eyeful, but the bottom line is: I don't want boys to see my daughter naked.

Now that Callie's found her Cho Cho, she's busted out of Eden with a vengeance. Her nakedness is now tinged with a hint of what's to come. Unlike Eve, Callie's thrilled with her new knowledge. How 'bout them apples, Serpent?

In a way that feels like spying, I spy. I check in with Callie's teacher; there's been no more squirming. Apparently the wooden chair was a one-night stand.

When Callie has a friend over and I notice her door's closed, I just happen to have an armload of her laundry to put away. Her stuffed animals are spread over the floor and they're playing Jungle Vet. Not Doctor, not Naked Jungle Vet. G-rated Jungle Vet.

It seems Callie's heeding my directions about privacy. She's not a Public Diddler.

But Callie still makes time to play with her Cho Cho alone. One night when Callie loiters in the tub, I vent to my husband.

"She's at it again. The water's cold and she won't get out."

"Just pull the plug."

"Honey, this is a balancing act. If we somehow give Callie the message to lock up her Cho until she's got a ring on her clitoris-twirling finger, she could end up repressed. Or, worse, she rebels and turns into the neighborhood tramp."

"Or we keep doing what we're doing, and she ends up fine."

I sigh. "I just so don't want to screw her up."

With as much gusto as a universal remote allows, he snaps off the TV.

"Look, I'm not thrilled about this Cho Cho thing either. But there's nothing wrong with Callie—"

"You're the one who said she's young to start diddling—"

"Well, she's started, so now we live with it. She doesn't in public, right?"

"Right, but—"

"—Stop! You're a good mother. A great mother. Quit overthinking; you'll get a handle on this."

"How do you know?"

"I just do."

"You're sure?"

He flicks SportsCenter back on. The daily highlights have just started. He offers me a swig of his beer, and I take a long, cold swallow.

"I have absolute faith in you." He wiggles his eyebrows suggestively. "Wanna see my Top Ten Plays of the Day?" He presses his cool, hopsy lips against mine. I lean into the kiss.

A shriek erupts from the bathroom.

"Mom-meeeeee!" It's Callie. "The water's freezing and I need a towel!"

My mother never worried about this stuff. In fact, she welcomed it. "I missed the sexual revolution," she announced countless times, "by one year. One measly year!" She's still bitter.

She encouraged me to tell her before I decided to "do it," so she could get me a diaphragm. She asked embarrassing questions about how much I knew, or didn't know, about anatomy. She commented on my menstrual cycles and my boobs, as if discussing the weather. "Your breasts are filling out, full and high. Why don't we shop for a B cup this weekend?"

She was so open and encouraging that I completely tuned her out.

When I was twelve, she overheard me and a girlfriend wondering whether a man could pee inside a woman when they were having sex. Mom hauled books off the shelf: wordy, illustrated books,

books with photographs, books with indices, for god's sake. She kept us captive for the longest twenty minutes of my life, explaining in detail why it was almost—but not entirely—impossible for an erect penis to urinate.

For some reason that girl never came back to my house. And I never asked my mom about sex. Who had that much time?

Since I want Callie to be comfortable talking to me about her body, I reject my mother's ultrainformative approach, which achieved the opposite effect with me. Neither can I blow it off as a normal milestone, despite my husband's absolute faith. How to achieve this delicate balance?

I consider my husband's advice to stop overthinking Callie's diddling. It isn't as if sex is on Callie's radar screen; she's only just discovered her Cho Cho. And, like Isaac Newton and gravity, she didn't really discover it, she just named something that had always been there.

I decide to take underthinking a step further and pretend there's nothing going on between Callie and her Cho Cho. To hell with delicate balance. Problems always go away when you ignore them, right?

After a week of intentional denial, the stars align for me and my husband to attempt marital-bed sex. We're both in bed and awake at the same time; the baby's in between feedings; no one's having nightmares or needs a glass of water; we both have the energy and desire.

We're getting right down to business when I catch myself generating a mental grocery list instead of an orgasm. I push my husband away.

"What's wrong?"

He asked for it. "I suddenly remembered that burned-out lightbulb in the hall. Which made me think about going to the hardware store. But what else do we need at the hardware store? A new lock for our bedroom door. Because any minute one of our kids will come bursting in on us and you'll have to pretend you're getting something out of my eye again. That made me think of how we skip foreplay and rush through sex all the time, and here we are finally doing it, and I'm thinking about lightbulbs."

He strokes my shoulder. "I'll fix the lock this weekend."

"It's not about the lock!"

"Shh!"

I hiss, "Down that dark hall, Callie's Cho Cho is waking up, and mine's in a coma."

He stares at me. "That's messed up," he says. "You sound . . . jealous."

"No! It's just, she's got all this fun ahead of her, and I'm— we're—" I can't say out loud, *we're stuck in rushed marital-bed sex mode*. I've already spoiled the moment.

Ignoring the issue isn't working. I'm back to seeking a delicate balance.

I don't feel like asking any of my friends or neighbors, "Hey, does your daughter diddle? Just wondering, 'cuz Callie's discovered her vagina and named it. Your daughter does that too, right?"

The Internet yields erratic results. "Most females begin masturbating at the onset of puberty," offers one dubious site. "And some never masturbate at all." Many more sites are blocked by our parental controls.

Maybe there's something helpful in one of those books my mother tried to press upon me. I pop into the neighborhood bookstore, but nothing in the parenting section appeals. As I breeze toward the exit, a title stops me in my tracks: *The Vagina Monologues,* by Eve Ensler.

That night I read *The Vagina Monologues* in one sitting. Then I read it again. Holy crap! There are women in weeping, joyous love with their vaginas, women who purposely disown their vaginas, singing vaginas, bad-luck vaginas, mythical vaginas. And so many names! There's "Itsy Bitsy," "fannyboo," and in one heartbreaking monologue, "coochi snorcher."

Compared to "coochi snorcher," "Cho Cho" sounds tame.

I kick myself for missing *The Vagina Monologues* on stage (couldn't get a sitter). Ensler transforms a word most people won't even say out loud into several distinct voices. Maybe if I initiate a discussion with Callie, starring Cho Cho in a nonsexual role, I'll nail that delicate balance.

It's time for a vagina dialogue with my daughter.

I need somewhere quiet and private to take this baby step with Callie. No such place exists in our home. It has to be the car.

I glance in the rearview mirror. Callie's contentedly watching the world slide past.

"Callie, if your vagina could wear clothes, what would it wear?"

When she stops laughing she answers straight-faced.

"Underwear, of course."

"And if your vagina could say two words, what would it say?"

"It would say, 'Gotta pee!'"

Of course. "One last question, Callie. Wait—do you really have to pee?"

"No, I was just answering the question."

"OK. The last question is, what does your vagina smell like?"

Again, hoots and giggles from the backseat. "I know what it smells like, because I just know, but I don't know how to say it in words. It just smells like a vagina."

These aren't the answers of a compulsive diddler; they're too practical. It dawns on me that Callie doesn't think of her Cho Cho in a romantic way. She's just engaging in scientific investigation. She isn't the type to consider her Cho Cho "a shell, a tulip, her destiny," as one of Eve Ensler's characters does—not that there's anything wrong with that. Perhaps this child will turn out fine, in spite of her overthinking mother.

Callie interrupts my thoughts.

"Why did you ask me those questions?"

"Well, Callie, I read a book. About women talking about their vaginas. And the woman who wrote the book asked a lot of women those three questions."

"Do you have any more questions to ask me?"

"Not really. She asked everyone those three, and then women told stories about their vaginas."

"Can I tell a story about my vagina?"

My grip on the steering wheel tightens.

"Sure."

"Once upon a time I was walking along and my vagina ripped itself off from my body and started walking with me."

Wow. Rough opener.

"But," continues Callie, "since vaginas don't have legs, it didn't really walk with me, it floated next to me."

I'm comforted. Floating's more pleasant than ripping.

"I couldn't hold its hand at the crosswalk, because vaginas don't have hands, either, so—wait a minute! Mom! Look at that puppy! It's sooo cute! Aw, Mom, can we get a puppy? Please?"

And just like that, we're off floating vaginas and on to Callie's latest cause, GetMeAPuppyNowOrIWillDie.Org, to which I refuse to pander until the baby is chewing steak, potty trained, and sleeping through the night in his own bed.

Callie's definitely gonna be OK.

Even with a coochi snorcher named Cho Cho.

The Dignity Channel

Jann Turner

Writing as Kit Thomas—the heroine
of her forthcoming novel
The Dignity Channel

I wish I could say that the best sex I ever had was this morning, but I didn't have sex this morning. I haven't had morning sex in years. As a matter of fact, I haven't had any kind of sex in a very, very long time. I don't like to think about that too much, after all I am thirty-nine years old, have great tits, a curvy body, and an above-average capacity for fun. I am supposed to be approaching the shimmering summit of my sexual appetite and energies—yet I have to concentrate to remember the details of when and how I last got laid.

I was at work. I had just pulled an all-nighter, finishing off the cuts on thirteen episodes of the Alpine Air series. I stood up from my computer as the sun rose, needing a cup of coffee. I was at the machine, pouring milk into a mug, when Ivan, the channel's head of development, stalked down the corridor. I leaned forward so my hair would obscure my face, hoping to avoid any kind of conversation. Not that he was in the habit of conversing with lowly editors, but just in case. Mercifully he walked straight past me. I peered up to watch his retreating back. His neck looked like it had been welded to his shoulders in an inflexible posture-perfect position, like the action hero dolls Jacqui and I played with when we were kids, because our mother and father disapproved of Barbie and Sindy as role models for their daughters. Ivan's body was very action hero but dressed in neatly pressed studentlike gear—jeans and a close-fitting cotton knit T-shirt with a pair of bright white Converse all stars. I was still staring, noticing how his hair curled outward from the nape of his neck, when he stopped and turned around. As if he'd just remembered something. Like my name.

He was a good ten, long-legged strides away down the corridor, looking straight at me. I froze, my hand cramping around the handle of the milk jug.

"It's Kit, right?" he said.

I nodded mutely.

"You vision mixed the pope's funeral," he stated in a tone that flatlined, like his eyes.

I nodded again. Ivan smiled, a gleaming, capped-tooth smile.

"Nice work," he said.

I frowned, wondering if he was being sarcastic. Ivan was not known for compliments. "Really?"

"Really," he affirmed, with a dip of his chin, and then he held out his arm, gesturing for me to walk ahead of him. "Come talk to me in my office." It was not an invitation.

This was unusual, to say the least. I hesitated, trying to read his expression for some clue as to whether or not I was about to be fired. His features gave nothing away; they were as plastic and as set as action man's, neither reproachful nor laudatory. So I put down the milk jug and did as he asked.

His office was vast, the same detergent bright white of the common areas and lesser offices at the Dignity Channel. I half expected someone in a lab coat to emerge from a secret door, as if we were in an ad for ethical pharmaceutical research. Against the back wall was a lean, low, chrome-legged white leather sofa facing toward floor-to-ceiling windows and a long narrow desk with a series of computer screens atop it, trailing streamers of wiring. Ivan's screens faced away from the view; I would have had it the other way around.

I heard the door closing and seconds later he materialized beside me; not touching, but standing very close to me.

"I love that river," he said. I looked up beyond the roof decks and water towers at the sun-dazzled stretch of the Hudson with its traffic of Circle Line cruisers and ships and barges and life going on and I felt like I was floating outside of a life, outside my skin. I shook my head in an attempt to shake the feeling out of me. He glanced over at me then strode toward his desk.

"Editors don't often see this view. You keep us locked up, away from any natural light," I said, straining for a light, humorous tone.

He pulled open a tiny drawer on his table. "Seems to me you like it that way," he responded dryly.

"Really? How would you know?" I answered, sounding more edgy than I'd intended, and I wanted to take the words back, but Ivan appeared unfazed.

"Am I wrong?" he asked. Something in the intensity of his stare made me think about this. No, he wasn't wrong. Darkness and shadows were precisely what I clung to.

He pulled a tiny envelope from the drawer, unfolded it, and shook out a pile of white powder on the glass surface of his desk. This was possibly the last thing I'd expected him to do, bar leaping through the window.

I watched as he cut two lines of coke on the glass. These were not like John's wonky lines that came in all sizes so you always wanted to be the first to snort because that way you wouldn't end up with the smaller share; Ivan's lines were perfectly even. Suddenly my mouth was watering. He offered me a rolled-up ten-dollar bill. I did the line in several starts. He snorted his in one clean move. Then he stroked his forefinger over the glass and rubbed the dust into his gum, his finger pushing up the flap of his upper lip.

"So, why am I here? Are you going to fire me?" I asked, with an awkward chortle.

He shook his head. "I'm going to fuck you," he said, his lips stretching in something approximating a smile.

"You mean right now?" I queried.

He nodded. But he made no move toward me. Instead he cut another pair of lines—these two fatter than the last. And once again he offered me the rolled-up note so that I could go first. I stepped toward him so that I could snort, and as I bent down he moved nearer. I could feel him so close that my hair stood on end with the electricity of his desire, though he wasn't touching me. He took the note when I was finished, but he didn't use it, instead he cleaned the glass with his forefinger and then pushed it between my lips, rubbing the coke against my gums and then my tongue.

I didn't move at all, not even to suck his finger, which is what I imagined he wanted. That would have been the raunchy thing to do. But the possible eroticism of his finger probing my mouth was pushed aside by the onrush of the drug, which I could feel prickling in my fingertips and charging into all the veins and tissues and sinews of me with the power of a flash flood. This time it rendered me speechless and motionless. It had been doing this all too often lately, paralyzing my limbs. Only my mind ran wild, like a frantic chicken that didn't understand the cause of its panic but knew that it must run, run, run. And my mind was running in ribbons of astonishment and pleasure and detachment and revulsion and confusion. Did he think I wanted him to fuck me? And my frantic chicken mind ran down the road of why would I want that? And then off down the road of yes, yes, that is so what I want and then no, it doubled back to the intersection of do I feel horny? Or don't I? I wasn't sure if I felt anything at all, at least not for him. And the chicken ran on and on and on. Even as he took me by my shoulders and turned me around and pushed in the small of my back so I was leaning forward and bracing my hands on the table as he deftly unbuttoned my fly and cold fingers touched my skin and slid my jeans and then my panties down my thighs, even then my chicken brain was running in pointless circles so that I was as acutely aware of the serifs in the typeface on the memorandum that was lying directly in front of me as I was of the rip of a condom packet and the fluttering fumble of his fingers as he got himself covered and then the rubbery thwack of his penis against my hip before he pushed himself into me.

And there was a part of me that was aroused by what he was doing. Or was it what we were doing? Though I wasn't doing very much as he thrust slowly in and then out of me, his breath hot on my neck and pulsing in my ear in an itchy sort of way. All I was doing was pressing my palms into the cold glass of the desktop, willing myself to feel more than I did, willing myself to feel more than fractionally aroused.

But I couldn't. And I didn't.

He came. Not too soon, but soon enough. I could feel the quiver of his ejaculation inside me. A series of small, animal grunts accompanied the shiver and then he was still. The grip of his fingers on my waist tightened, but he didn't fall against me, didn't hold me, and didn't pretend to any kind of intimacy, although there was a gentlemanly consideration in the way he pulled out of me. Then he was quick to dispose of the condom and to pull his pants back up and to bend once again to the task of cutting lines. "I like your work," he said.

I resigned the next day.

That's not the kind of sex I want to remember. Though it's cer-

tainly not the worst sex I've ever had. My list of worst-evers is probably much like that of most other woman of my age, a labia-shrivelling
inventory that's best saved in the "forgotten" file. There was the
holiday romance who jumped me several times a night, hammered
at me like a jackrabbit for a couple of minutes before emitting a loud
squeak, then rolling off and back into sleep—nothing to write home
about. There was the confident guy at the company retreat—the
gregarious jock who seemed to promise a big, swinging dick but
couldn't get it up, and when at last he did—after hours of patient
soothing and coaxing of both ego and prick—ejaculated in a miserable little squirt on the bedclothes before he'd managed to get his
penis anywhere near me. Then there's the guy who fucked me for
hours on a kudu skin ottoman in front of a blazing fire, but in the
light of subsequent information the whole scene had to be regraded
from sensational to seedy. Turned out my long-endurance lover
had been brutally cuckolded and the house of the blazing fire and
the ottoman would soon belong to his soon-to-be ex-wife and her
new man. It never feels good to have been party to someone else's
revenge fuck; he might as well have been humping the kudu.

Curiously, good sex, for me, doesn't require a postmortem—
like an obviously natural death. Bad sex, on the other hand, involves
a mandatory inquest, conducted by a friend and myself over coffee
in the days following the event. Bad sex is something I blame—at
least in my spoken testimony—on my partner in the crime. The
truth, of course, is that it takes two to tango, and the success of
the steps not only depends on grace and consideration of the indi-
viduals concerned but also is—crucially—a function of the dynamic
between the dancers.

My married friends often ask me, with the hunger of deprivation
in their eyes, for details of my latest encounter. As if my single life is
a series of episodes in an adult rom com, to be devoured vicariously
in the sexual desert of marital bliss. Truth is that when there is sex,

it is often just middling, which—like a meal that's not terrible, but not delicious either—always leaves the taste of disappointment on the tongue.

There have been promising instances that turned into fun sex. One of my most surprising flirtations ever popped up at the second-time-around wedding of my cousin Pearl. My seducer was twenty-two years old, the son of Pearl's best friend—her bridesmaid on this occasion. He was a tall, blue-eyed, tousle-haired blond. And he was almost half my age. Too young for me to have taken note of him, which is probably why he made it his business to introduce himself to me before the service, told me how sexy I looked as he swirled past me carrying his mother's confetti basket. I thought he was joking, but I thanked him. Sometimes even fake flattery feels good. Turned out he wasn't joking at all. Later, when the reception was in full swing and the party was frilled out on sparkling wine, he took me by the hand, marched me down to the parking lot, pushed me against a car and bit onto my lower lip, sucked on it hard, and then slid his tongue into my mouth. Within seconds we were semi-naked. He was hard as rock candy and as hyperactive as a toddler on ice cream. He seemed to think I'd be disappointed if he didn't display an advanced knowledge of the entire Kama Sutra. As if he had to perform like some character in a porno. Perhaps that's what I was to him, some character in a porno—the older woman, his very own Mrs. Robinson. He was so busy positioning and repositioning us that he didn't come. I did—despite the complex entanglement of our limbs and the discomfort in my knees and elbows. I came deliciously.

That was delightful, but I wouldn't call it great sex. Certainly not the best sex ever.

My friend Ian says the best sex he has ever had was with a guy whose last name he doesn't know and whom he meets once in a while at a cruising spot near Bethesda Fountain. For Ian the essential ingredient is fun. His Central Park sex toy really enjoys him— not like a fussy gourmand showing off the exquisite subtlety and range of his sexual tastes—but like a hungry youth who eats him up with gusto and generosity and simple pleasure.

My friend Ida loves sex with strangers. Relationships are not her thing. The last time she was dating someone and I asked her how it was going she said—"He phones me every day. It gives me the creeps." Recently she signed on with one of the big Internet dating sites. She advertised for a man who wanted a regular physical relationship without emotional commitment, making it plain that she was looking for a fuck buddy—not a boyfriend or a husband. Within hours she was inundated with responses. Most of the respondents were married men who were also looking for sex uncomplicated. She arranged to meet a selection of seven for interviews. The interview was conducted—in each case—over cappuccinos in the Barnes & Noble on Union Square. The initial seven were whittled down to four, who were granted physical tryouts, which were conducted in a hotel room, the cost shared. Two contenders emerged. The favorite and the ultimate champion was a married doctor who declared up front that he adored his wife, loved his kids, had no desire to upset his home life, but needed more sex—he and his wife hadn't done it in a decade.

And so—every Wednesday at 5:45 P.M.—Ida has an appointment with the doctor at his consulting rooms. She wears exotic underwear and he opens up his drawer of toys. He has introduced her to slipper spanking, ostrich feather ticklers, and some light whipping. He courteously ensures that she comes at least once before he goes for his own climax. They talk a little before and after, but not much. The point is to fuck, not to make friends.

Much as I'd like it to, that wouldn't work for me. That's because my mind and my clitoris are connected by a horribly complex tangle of tensions and triggers. Great sex is obviously a matter of taste, determined by what it is you're looking for on a spectrum ranging from transcendent emotional intimacy to a physical workout with an orgasmic ending. The height of pleasure for me falls somewhere in between. Sex as mind fuck, heart attack, and clitoral firestorm. A triple-connect of head, heart, and loin. A total sensory sundae.

It's hard to describe great sex; it's so sacred, so private when it's good. It is of that order of existence and action that is beyond words—greater and grander than anything that can be distilled in sentences. That's why written descriptions of wonderful sex often end up sounding cheesy or silly. So I'm not going to describe this at length, you'll have to take my word for it—my best sex ever was with the man I married.

We met at college. We were young and we plummeted ecstatically into love; making love whenever and wherever we could, not because it was transgressive, but because it was urgently necessary. It was a total exploration of the other, a drenching of the senses, a total immersion in scent, taste, touch, seat, skin sound, breath. Every millimeter of his being had to be experienced, just as every millimeter of mine was touched and tasted and adored. It was utter; there was nothing else—no past, no future, simply the moment and one another—both completely exposed, painfully vulnerable and completely fearless.

More than a decade later we were divorced, but I'll never forget that first time, in Luke's dorm room at Yale, in a single bed that fitted us amply because our bodies fit so perfectly and so close. It was the first time that I came. Afterward he ran a bath in the communal change rooms, and together, wrapped in towels, we skittered up the cold staircase into the cubicle and soaked in silence in the deep, hot water. With his warm flannel he washed my face and my neck and my breasts and my belly—our eyes smiling, wide open and locked on one another.

Miss Honeypot Marries

A Short Story

Barbara Victor

From the time she was aware of sex in her imagination, each act in her fantasy was perfect, the best sex she ever had, the next time always more incredibly delicious than the time before. All the dashing men who were friends of her father's, husbands and lovers of the women who were close to her mother, taught her about seduction. The moguls, actors, writers, doctors, lawyers, painters, diplomats, the men who came to swim and play tennis in the country or who sipped cocktails at parties in the city, made her aware of the "it" her friends giggled and whispered about. "Did she do it?" "I heard she did it." "Did he try to do it?"

By the time her teenage years were winding down, she was way beyond the "it." She understood the subtle glances of the sophisticated and suave older men, the light touch on her arm to help her on with a coat, the words that held double meanings to camouflage the message, the embarrassed glances when she dared to look them in the eye, the flicker of hope when she hugged them too close. Because she understood their silent language, she knew why Eddie left Debbie for Liz and Frank left Nancy for Ava, and Archie secretly preferred Veronica though he always stayed safely with Betty. At sixteen and seventeen, she even understood what Hammett saw in Hellman, how Monroe desired Miller, and Bogart and Bacall exploded on the screen.

The "it" had no form or memory, no aftermath of regret or embarrassment, as it remained elusive and intangible, created and orchestrated by her alone—masturbation with a willing partner who was under her control and direction. Miss Honeypot was the Alexander Haig of sexual fantasy. "I am in charge here" was her mantra. Those older men were all Cary Grant, obliged to recite words written for them by her, succumb when the script called for surrender, retreat when the director, her again, needed sexual tension.

She had sex before she had sex. She had great sex before she ever had bad sex.

Miss Honeypot's abstinence was never based on lack of daring or fear of reprisal but rather on a dread of disappointment that would contradict the perfection of making love that went beyond her brain. There were good girls and bad girls and somewhere in her mind, until she could come out and be both, the bad girl hidden within the good girl, until she could find someone who would understand that fantasy was her game, she was out of the running. Her desire was the chase that ended in half-finished acts which always promised more and better and best. Hunting for the drama that would turn into ecstasy impelled her to seek out the perfect candidates to share an actual foray into bed. The "it" became the "what if" when the first kiss at sixteen with a brooding, tragic boy who died two years later by his own hand, kept her going for another two years until at eighteen, the "what if" became a "so what" when the son of a literary giant tricked her into believing that knowing the steps of the dance standing up had bearing on the moves lying down. A black lace party dress ripped down the back was a remnant of his misplaced enthusiasm, lipstick askew covering a bruised lip happened more out of anger than ardor, which made the whole encounter off the charts and impossible to rank. She was his Lolita in the flesh. Coupling with him was a trip to a zoo where wild animals roamed free and which had her scurrying back to the safety of untried yet fulfilling fantasies. After doing "it" for years with happy endings, she made the mistake of doing "it" for real. The scale from worst to best had taken form.

In her twenties, Tuscany melted her heart and an Italian opera singer melted her icy veneer. Miss Honeypot heard him sing before the world sang his praises. He was the perfect panacea for her second encounter of the intimate kind and the appropriate send-off before heading down a Swiss slope into the arms of a married mogul who gave her a ride on his private plane. From there to Belgrade and the impoverished Yugoslav student who had no bathroom or shower in his room in the shabby pension, but who offered lilac soap to bathe in his sink. The affair was sweet and tender but geographically impossible, which was why it seemed great for the seventeen hours that they tangled. By then, the impossible, improbable, and highly unlikely freed her to hit and run.

On a train headed for Paris, she considered her position on the scale from worst to best. For a brief instant she had great though in reality, she was still firmly on worst, hoping to inch her way up to passable.

Driving along the quai in Paris at dusk where rooftops cut magical designs in the sky, she heard *the* question for the first time. "Am I the best you ever had?" Best? With the exception of seventeen hours of silent sex with an impoverished Yugoslav, she had just gotten over worst, passable was barely possible and adequate was a distant dream. The man asking *the* question was French and adept at food and wine, which, in her state of confusion, had her comparing him to the rich risotto she had devoured in Tuscany with the thin Nouveau Beaujolais that she had just tasted and despised. Too young to be so embittered, Miss Honeypot headed home to America with the intention of burying herself in work. While buried, she married a grim but brilliant economist who baffled her with his choice of monetary policy and his penchant for serial infidelity with obese women who lived in trailers. If fantasy was still her mantra, gratitude was obviously his. Sex with him was neither bad nor good, neither best nor worst. It was married missionary mundane and monotonous. While she wrote copy in her head for the news broadcast the following evening, he toiled away at intercourse. He was Portnoy. She was liver. Once in Berlin with him, she wrote a postcard to her mother. "Who is this man who calls himself my husband, and what is his name doing on my passport?"

Back in New York, divorced and working in television, Miss Honeypot met them all. There were the men who flattered, chased, pursued, begged, threatened, abused, drank, drugged, and sometimes even made it past passable. There was the anchor who used toys, the Greek who used drugs, and the producer who used the 8h13 back to Scarsdale to excuse his premature ejaculation. Another husband followed, a man whose face she couldn't quite place years after the divorce when they crossed paths at an airport.

Something clicked in her brain. Bad sex was easy to recognize. Good sex, though elusive, was tough. It had little to do with technique, size, durability, or improbability. It had only to do with finding a man who had her number.

Settled in New York, and working in television, the dashing older men who were still her father's friends were a decade more cynical, less confident and suddenly willing to risk it. It was a match made in Greek mythological heaven. They needed to assure their own immortality. She was Electra let loose in a geriatric ward. Her thirties were a blur of whirlwind encounters with men whose desire for her took precedent over her own sexual pleasure, when her body was taut and her power at its apex, when her ability to seduce gave her the right to go careening in the wrong direction down a one-way street. The scale from worst to best was all about conquest and some bizarre need to rebel against her roots. Had she been Catholic, her target would have been a priest. Had she been daring, it would have been a woman. Had she been in Auschwitz, it would have been a Nazi. Her story was banal. It was fear that propelled her to choose the worst and convince herself that she had found the best.

Fantasy is delicious. Reality is rarely better. Then it happened. For the first time, reality was the fantasy Miss Honeypot had never had.

Somewhere in her midthirties, she found herself floundering professionally and personally, convinced that she had hit the bottom, certain that the best was behind her and the future was bleak. Halfway down that one-way street, Miss Honeypot collided with a man. He was handsome, adorable, funny, guilt ridden, grief stricken, frightened, professionally in limbo, exiting a marriage, and the new father of an infant. At first glance, he was everything she wanted and everything she feared. Had he asked what her astrological "sign" was, she would have said "available," but he only asked her name, where she lived, and what she did. The first two questions were easy to answer. The third was like an arrow piercing her heart. No longer able to hide behind a glamorous job, bored by men who had never penetrated her soul, desperate to regain some semblance of sanity and order in her life, Miss Honeypot fell madly in love, albeit with the unspoken but conditional proviso, "enter at your own risk." He did. She did. Within twenty minutes or so, they were living together. It was the best sex she ever had. It was the best love she ever had. It was the funniest, most intellectually challenging time she ever had. It was the most tender and exciting moment in her life. And she and he did everything in their power to turn heaven into hell.

Their fights were an exercise in linguistics and psychoanalysis. His command of the language equaled or even surpassed hers. His ability to dissect her motives and machinations destroyed the little power she had left. He had her number to the point where he knew her body, defenses, and games, and could even dismantle her armor with nothing more lethal than his tongue. Their routine was predictable. They made love all night. Who knew what Miss Honeypot was capable of doing with a man who knew what he was doing? Starved at dawn, they stumbled to a neighborhood diner for food, came home and made themselves presentable to show up either to work or to interview for work. In the evening, he came home, carrying a shoulder bag on one arm and his infant in the other. His dog was a big part of their life until they parted and the dog jumped out a window. They would never know if it was suicide or dementia or perhaps sadness that the perfect couple had simply given up. When they parted officially and her closets were emptied of his clothes, her shelves bare of his books, her bathroom devoid of his toiletries, he took up residence in a building next door. He could see her come and go though never for a moment did she ever imagine he cared enough to suffer. She watched him come and go, steeling herself against the pain of missing him by taking to her bed or diligently plotting her next professional move. Six months went by and he saw other women, many women, not particularly plausible women, while she dated the occasional man. They had their moments. He would call. Miss Honeypot would answer. They would make mad passionate love and know that the bond wasn't broken but the fear was too overwhelming to give it another try. He would tell her that all she had to do was ask. She would respond that if only he would say what he wanted. And it went on like that for several years—until she got a job and moved to Paris, and he found a woman and made a new life.

Based in Paris and working for a major news magazine, her job took her to the Middle East where the reality of love was quick and impersonal, death lurking at every bedpost, bombs flashing in the distance through shattered windows. It was essential to be dressed at all times as militias attacked the hotel in Beirut where the foreign press stayed. Evacuation could be imminent. The guys who covered the wars were expert at in-and-out. She was expert at running for the story. She had no time or desire for furtive moments. She lived with her boots on, her notepad and pen handy (no outlets on the battlefield), ready to rock and roll to a safe place behind the Green Line, after the usual television questions about how it feels to be the sole survivor of a massacre. In Beirut, where war raged and the bouquet of terror armies was as varied as petals thrown on a funeral pyre at a Hindu cremation, Miss Honeypot lost her sense of fantasy. Those same male colleagues, who wore trench coats and safari jackets, smoked unfiltered cigarettes, and expertly handled a Swiss Army knife, were considered the real thing. They were the war correspondents, the swaggering macho men who, backdropped by the ravaged scenery of devastation and destruction, did their five-minute standups in all the horrific corners of the Middle East. She was the only woman. Sex under fire was an unimaginable fantasy. Bombs crashing, grenades exploding, sporadic gunfire surrounding tangled bodies in fields where land mines were suspected, pushed the mercury up on the thermometer from passable to good to great to nothing after the moment ended.

What did she know that they had not yet learned? What had she forgotten that they would never know?

One thing Miss Honeypot knew for certain about her male colleagues was that beneath the belted trench coats, waiting for Moses to hand them the Ten Commandments at the foot of Mount Sinai, the smaller the penis, the more they bragged and boasted and described in detail what they had done in the mine fields.

One thing she learned was that men like that didn't have scales from worst to best. It was sex—yes or no—and they moved in like a one-man army, exterminating villages before careening onto the next helpless civilian enclave, a notch in their belts or on the butts of their Uzis that counted the number of bodies—dead or alive.

For the first ten years while Miss Honeypot lived and worked in Paris, she embraced celibacy with a vow as fierce as a nun's. In her forties, time had been kind enough to make her vocal position on abstinence a challenge to the new crop of macho journalists, insipid French intellectuals, the up-and-coming new generation of moguls, and those same impoverished students who had since become destitute artists and writers. Days after her fiftieth birthday, she met the perfect man—an impotent and powerful French politician who offered a respectable base as she traveled around Europe and the Middle East covering the same old internecine struggles and terror attacks.

Ten years into their relationship and beginning her second decade in Paris, Miss Honeypot happened to be in New York, finishing a book and refurbishing her parents' apartment while they were in Palm Beach. Life had changed. They were old. Her mother was ill. Her father was desperate to make her well. An e-mail arrived from her agent. He had forwarded a message from the only man in her life that she had loved, along with a cynical remark at the end that read, "Another one has come out of the woodwork."

The man had not exactly "come out of the woodwork." They had been in touch on and off throughout the years, though she hadn't talked to him for a while. On that occasion, she replied immediately. He called. She answered. He told her he had a dream on the eve of his sixty-fifth birthday. He had to find her. He invited her for lunch. Miss Honeypot said she didn't eat lunch. What about dinner? He said it was difficult, as he had recently married. Why call? Why now? Why me? He was the age his father was when he died. He wanted a real life with the love of his life.

They met for dinner and the years disappeared. She knew then what she had never known or never dared to believe. Somehow she had entered his psyche and owned his soul, and for twenty-something years he had harbored a hope that would not go away. When he kissed her on the street after dinner, she was surprised by her words. "You awakened me." They saw each other every day while she was in New York. Approaching sixty, it was unthinkable to take off her clothes and make love with a stranger. But he was no stranger. She knew his body as well as her own. To him, her body hadn't changed since they had first met when she was somewhere in her midthirties. He still had her number but, by then, she had her number too, as well as his. They went slowly, considering the passion and intensity of their feelings, aware that there was no room to turn heaven into hell this time around.

When she returned to Paris, they spoke four or five times a day, e-mailed constantly and made plans to do what had to be done to pick up where they had left off. Four months later, she was living with him in New York. He was in the throes of divorce and she had packed up her life in Paris.

In the beginning, back then, they made love constantly to calm the anxiety and guilt and pain of what they knew was a trail of bruised and battered bodies they had left behind. They struggled to find their place with each other. They laughed at their sheer insanity to think they could pull this off after middle age. They sparred. They fought. They laughed. They cried. Sex wasn't even an issue. It was the least of their struggles. It was amazing, surprising, unpredictable, never the same, always new, and doing things that they never dared to do with anyone before. Sex was suddenly more than doing "it." It was trust. It was nurturing and caring love. It was the fact that a woman of sixty had a man who still saw her as she was when she was young. It was the fact that a man in his mid-sixties had a woman who saw the only man she had ever loved evolve into a grown-up who had conquered the demons that had haunted him the last time around.

They got married. Miss Honeypot married Mr. Intensity. Miss Celibate married Mr. Promiscuous.

Best Sex Ever

A Systematic Review with Meta-Analysis

Jessica Winter

Objective

The aim of this longitudinal case study was a qualitative determination of best practice in sexual intercourse and affiliated activities (referred to hereafter as "relations") for a thirty-two-year-old female (hereafter the "primary subject"). The study reviewed both uncontrolled data (collected over a seven-year period) and controlled data (collected over a thirty-day period) to assess methods for maximum optimization of physical and emotional affect during relations.

Background

Though there is no clinically accepted definition of sexual best practice, criteria generally incorporate permutations of location (and novelty thereof[a]), posture (and novelty thereof[b]), overall

---

a. See data collected by the subjects in the woodlands of Bures, Suffolk, England, reviewed in *The Incident at Arger Fen* (2003).
b. See subjects' data reviewed in *The Diagnostics of the Diagonal; or, Meditations on the Gräfenberg Spot* (2002–present).

novelty[c], chronology, and quantitative data (measuring duration of action, outcome, and postcoital drop in IQ). Even anecdotally derived definitions are understood to be fluid, due to an evolving marketplace of instructional and/or performance-enhancing videos, books, articles, fitness regimens, grooming techniques, surgical interventions, visualization exercises, supportive footwear, dental modifications, aromatherapeutic houseplants, pedagogical séances, rain dances, ritual feasts, and other goods and services designed to facilitate best practice.

METHODS AND DESIGN

With the input of her long-term research collaborator, a forty-year-old male (hereafter the "secondary subject"), the primary subject accessed a range of performance-enhancing goods and services in three categories during the thirty-day experimental period: (1) audiovisual aids, in which compensated performers demonstrate techniques for best practice; (2) instructional literature, which provides textual and pictorial recommendations for best practice; and (3) "coregasm" exercises, which target muscles engaged in optimal completion of relations.

OUTCOMES

1. Audiovisual aids

Subjects reviewed audiovisual aids recommended for sustained clinical efficacy by the staff at Babeland, a retailer of technology-driven solutions for optimizing relations. Preliminary findings suggest that the subjects' association of best practice with crite-

---

c. See data collected by the subjects in Amsterdam, the Netherlands, reviewed in *They Came in through the Bathroom Window* (2003).

ria such as privacy[d], seclusion[e], and being-in-time contra-indicates spectatorship of relations that are mediated by the cinematographic apparatus. Researchers hypothesized that excessive exposure to audiovisual aids may create an alienation effect[f] whereby each partner becomes a critical (or "outside") observer and/or consumer of an intimate (or "inside") experience.[g] This critical distancing was evident in the subjects' improvised nomenclature for a noteworthy female performer's range of vocalizations, including "Sheep on Horseback," "Goat with Hernia," "Cow in Massage Chair," and "Liza Minnelli Gets a Bikini Wax."

However, between five and twenty minutes' exposure to audiovisual aids did nonetheless catalyze subjects' desire for relations, even if this exposure did not necessarily catalyze desire for further audiovisual aids. Thus, research indicates that an audiovisual aid *per se,* even or especially when abandoned before its conclusion, can prompt broadly imitative behavior and therefore effect optimized relations.

---

d. It should be noted that sound privacy is generally accepted to have a weaker correlation with optimized relations than visual privacy. See *Inadequate Hotel Soundproofing as Deterrent to Intimate Activities*: *An Opposing Viewpoint* (2003; updated 2004, 2006, 2008) and *When the Bedroom Overlooks a Courtyard*: *An Etiquette Guide for Couples* (2006; editions updated annually).

e. It should be noted that studies have found a direct, perhaps paradoxical, correlation between the aphrodisiac qualities of seclusion and the precariousness thereof. For further discussion, see *The Incident at Arger Fen.*

f. The original German term for this phenomenon, coined by playwright Bertolt Brecht, is *Verfremdungseffekt*, which is as sexy as it sounds.

g. The British popular rock band Pulp memorably dramatized the *Verfremdungseffekt* of what may be termed "pornographied" sex in its 1998 longplay album *This Is Hardcore*: "I've seen this storyline / Played out so many times before / That goes in there / Then that goes in there / Then that goes in there / Then that goes in there / And then it's over." Perhaps surprisingly, subjects do not find *This Is Hardcore* itself to exhibit an alienating effect on relations.

2. Instructional literature

Subjects reviewed a range of recently published instructional literature recommended for sustained clinical efficacy via Amazon.com
rankings and algorithms. Preliminary findings suggest that the subjects' association of best practice with criteria such as spontaneity
and improvisation[h] contraindicates the arguably overdetermined
nature of the selected prescriptive texts, which included role-
playing simulations ("Basically, one of you is a virgin/alien and
has no idea what sex is. The other person has to explain what they
should do"[i]), directives for inventory management ("Make a list of
ten things you want more of in bed, ten things you want less of, and
ten new things you'd like to try"[j]), and elaborate taxonomy ("G-Spot
Jiggy," "Rainbow Arch," "Lock and Load"[k]).

Pictorial recommendations were marginally more practicable.
Of the two sampled positions not yet enacted by the subjects over
the aforementioned seven-year period of uncontrolled data collection, the first position was clinically determined to have inhibitory
associations with exigencies occasioned by hiking and/or camping
trips lacking in lavatorial facilities. The second position was clinically determined to be extremely awesome.

Overall, subjects' response to instructional literature largely op-
erated according to a transitive property: Reading the texts inspired
attempts at best practice, but these attempts did not necessarily
accommodate the instructions contained in the texts (*viz.,* para-
normal ideations, produce- and condiment-focused shopping lists,
construction of Rainbow Arches). Thus, research indicates that

---

h. For further discussion, see *The Incident at Arger Fen.*
i. Elisabeth Wilson, *52 Brilliant Ideas—Great Sex: Bigger, Better, Faster, More*
(Perigree, 2008).
j. Tracey Cox, *Supersex* (Dorling Kindersley, 2009).
k. Christine Evans and David Usher, *101 Chocolate Sex Positions: With an Ultimate Safe Sex Guide for Guaranteed Satisfaction at Any Age and Shape*
(Self-Help Publishers, 2008).

an instructional book *per se,* even or especially when abandoned before its conclusion, can prompt broadly imitative behavior and therefore effect optimized relations.

3. *"Coregasm" exercises*

Primary subject reviewed and followed a range of online instructions for exercises recommended for sustained clinical efficacy via Google search. Exercises largely consisted of leg lifts (performed from a lying or suspended position) intended to strengthen and excite the lower-abdominal and pelvic-floor muscles, and also comprised "suspension yoga" positions performed in coordination with a sling-and-pulley system that retails online for $195 plus shipping and handling. Whilst these exercises did provoke the pleasurable tension and quasi-frustration associated with progression toward climax, the primary subject failed to experience an actual "coregasm" in the clinical research setting, unlike previous investigators.[1]

It should be noted, however, that this section of the study presented unique methodological challenges, as the primary subject would often feel overwhelmingly compelled to return to her place of residence before exercises were well under way, citing "personal matters" that required immediate resolution with the secondary subject. Thus, research indicates that a coregasm workout *per se,* even or especially when abandoned before its conclusion, can prompt broadly imitative behavior and therefore effect optimized relations.

---

1. An anonymous "coregasm" researcher quoted on MensHealth.com: *"Bam—* it hit me like a ton of bricks. I just stopped right then and there, got all pale in the face, and then busted out laughing. Everyone in the place was looking at me."

DISCUSSION

In formulating this project, the subject unwittingly placed herself and the secondary subject within a consumerist-managerial context: "consumerist" in that goods and services were accessed for the purposes of optimizing relations; and "managerial" in that relations were submitted to goal-setting and performance review. After extensive further inquiry, including a close reading of the "commodity fetish" entry on Wikipedia, it was determined that conflation of libidinous consumerism with the libido itself is inadvisable because it beckons market forces and affiliated hazards such as status anxiety and hyper-acquisitiveness into a nonprofit inner sanctum. Subjects risk casting relations in terms roughly equivalent to a PowerPoint presentation on the Kama Sutra featuring anatomical flowcharts and live accompaniment by Paris Hilton and Donald Trump atop a faux-marble conference table, with the lights on.

Subjects' brief and incomplete foray into the sexual-optimization marketplace was valuable, however, in reaffirming their commitment to a vigorous frontier spirit of inquiry and experimentation in pursuing best practice. This highly variable approach privileges the anticipation of the act as much as the act itself, and is especially vital as a complement to the devotional exclusivity of an optimized long-term collaboration.[m]

CONCLUSION

The best sex the subjects ever had is the sex they're having next.

---

m. *Viz.*, "I need you more than want you, and I want you for all time." Jimmy Webb, quoted in Glen Campbell, "Wichita Lineman" (1968).

Cock of My Dreams

A Graphic Fantasy

Marisa Acocella Marchetto

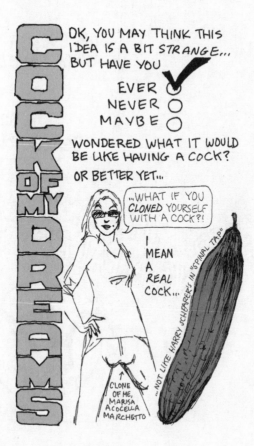

YOU KNOW HOW SCHOOLBOYS IN LOCKER ROOMS SHOW OFF HOW HUNG THEY ARE? WELL IF I HAD A CLONE WITH A COCK, MY/HER? ROD WOULD BE SO BIG, I/SHE'D? BE ABLE TO HANG...

NOT A TOWELETTE...

...OR A HAND TOWEL...

...OR EVEN A BATH TOWEL...

...BUT A BEACH TOWEL.

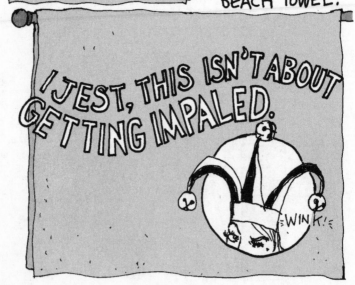

I JEST, THIS ISN'T ABOUT GETTING IMPALED.

=WINK!=

DON'T GET ME WRONG, IT'S NOT THAT I'M
TAKING MEN OUT OF THE EQUATION, I'M
JUST TALKING ABOUT LOCATION. FOR INSTANCE,
WHAT DO THEY LOVE EVEN *MORE* THAN
ASKING FOR DIRECTIONS?

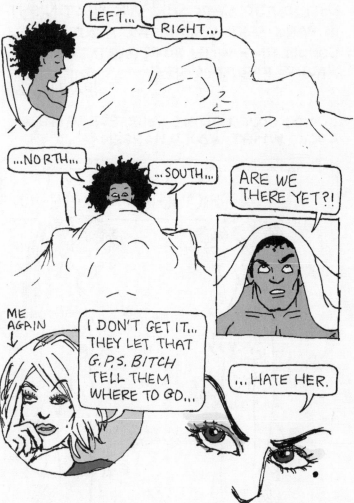

OF COURSE, HAVING A CLONE WITH A COCK
COULD *NEVER* REPLACE THE I JUST BEAT
CANCER SEX! WE JUST GOT MARRIED SEX!
I JUST GOT A DIVORCE SEX! I MADE A
MILLION DOLLARS SEX! OUR FIRST NIGHT
IN PARIS SEX! WHICH IS ALL ABOUT
CONNECTING WITH YOUR PARTNER AND
HAVING FABULOUS SEX!   BUT...

IF YOU COULD CLONE YOURSELF WITH A
COCK, WHAT WOULD HAPPEN?

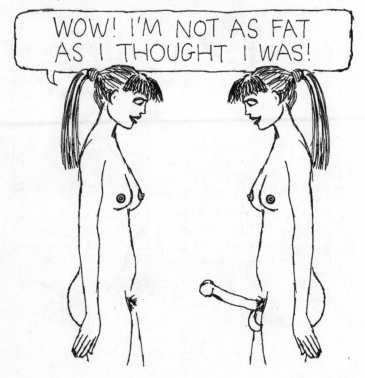

EITHER WAY, YOU ALWAYS COME FIRST!
IT'S A WIN-WIN! AFTERALL, WHO KNOWS
YOU BETTER THAN YOU KNOW YOURSELF?

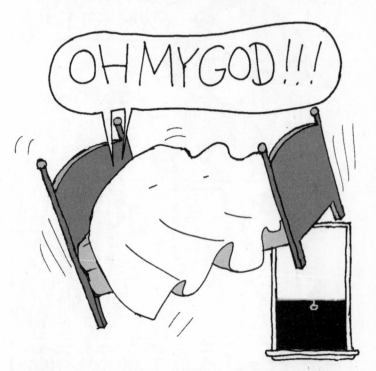

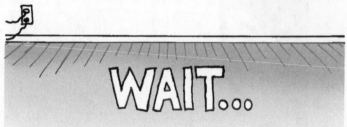

...AND HERE'S THE BEST PART...

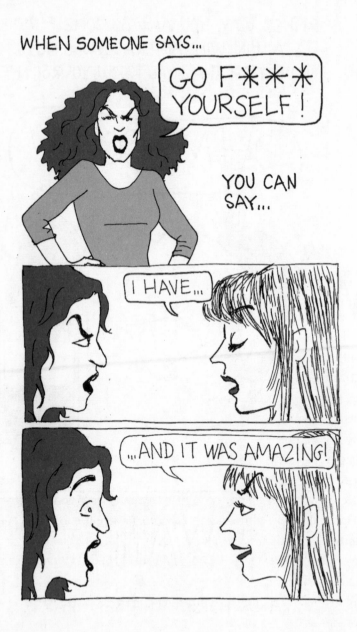

Cramming It All In

A Satire

Susan Kinsolving

We were madly, multiculturally, in love. We were habitually, historically, in heat.

He was my Peking Man; I was his fire. He was my wheel; I was his box. He called me his Demeter, Earth Mother, Cybele, Isis, and Corn Goddess. I was silk; he was silage.

To my giggling Greek girl, he was a gigantic Gilgamesh. He was Casanova; I feigned Chastity. He was Incubus to my Succubus, Benedict to my Beatrice, an otolaryngologist to my Deep Throat.

Every night, he showed me more of his special collections: codpieces, chastity belts, Valentines, dildos, and pre-Columbian stirrup-spout vessels.

He read Homer aloud, explaining etymologies without apologies for: androgyny, aphrodisiac, eroticism, hermaphroditism, nymphomania, and satyriasis. He quoted from Ovid's *Ars Amatoria,* the Kama Sutra, *Master Jung-ch'eng's Principles, Thy Neighbor's Wife, Couples, Fear of Flying,* and *Dog Breeding for Dummies.*

In the pink shell of my perfumed ear, he would whisper Sumerian songs asking "to put a hot fish in my naval."

Never erring with Eros, he was my guy; I was his gyne. He was a boy in my brothel, a powerhouse to pudenda, a yang to yin. He followed the advice of Master Tung-hsüan, working his Jade Stalk and Gamboling Wild Horses to my Cinnabar Cleft and Hovering Butterflies. He was a master without Masters & Johnson; kinky without Kinsey.

He also performed as a troubadour and jongleur, creating his own court, where I was the unconsummated lady and he, the chivalrous crusader. He was Lancelot to my Guinevere. How he could polish armor, night after knight, I never knew.

Sometimes he had me wear a blood bandage. Other times, he celebrated ancient circumcision rites, but never made the cut. Marvelously, he masqueraded as the Marquis, without inflicting much misery. He also played a dashingly devilish Donald Duck to my besotted Betty Boop. On a weekly basis, he celebrated The Rites of Spring.

Romance and dogma, sacred and profane, concessions and caricatures, all those made him someone extraordinary. He was the best; eventually, I was bested.

Now only memory brings back that final night with a full moon, swelling sea, and his sudden, spectacular vasocongestion. We were in systolic acceleration. His Cowper's gland opened, moistening and meeting my Bartholin's. His face grimaced, toes curled, and feet arched. His skin flushed. My brain was swamped and seared with sensation, like a superabundant sneeze coming on. Then came that seismic shocker with extravagant pyrotechnics. His cries resembled an ecstatic orangutan, an animalistic outpouring, a big O of inhuman annunciation, wild whoops. I fell silent. And then, a sweat broke out, and it all was over. Over with a big O.

I can only wonder where he went, and what it all meant, when he left without a word. Instead of a note, I found a box of condoms. I am keeping it, a memento, for our love child, when he comes of age.

Reticence and Fieldwork

Min Jin Lee

In 1995 when I was twenty-six years old, I quit my job as a corporate lawyer to write fiction full- time. Less than a year later, I had a fat book manuscript with a lofty title and an agent willing to send it out. Around the same time, I also asked my husband to read it. By then, Christopher and I had been married for about three years, and one of the reasons I fell in love with him was that he was a very good reader. The fact that he read Kobo Abe, Julian Barnes, and Wallace Stegner had been as important to me as his engaging sense of humor.

It took him a while to finish, but when he finally did, I asked him to be truthful.

"I didn't like your main character Annie. She's dull and unsympathetic. And there's no sex in the book."

My normally calm husband was nervous, and he didn't say anything more. If I didn't want the man I loved and respected to say these things, it was clear that he didn't enjoy saying them either. Within weeks, every major publisher had rejected my manuscript. I asked my agent to stop circulating it and buried the box of pages on the bottom shelf.

Over the years, as I worked on two other novel manuscripts

and a passel of short stories, Christopher's comments continued to buzz in my head, especially what he'd said about the lack of sex in the pages. Not every book needed to have sex in it, I argued with myself. That said, for most of my reading life, I'd been in thrall to late-nineteenth-century and early-twentieth-century classics with romantic plots and passionate heroines. The depictions of lovemaking in those books may seem quaint to the turn-of-the-twenty-first-century reader, but their sexual plots were outrageous for their respective times, even testing obscenity laws: Emma Bovary had a tryst in a horse-drawn carriage; George Eliot's dairymaid Hetty Sorrel was deflowered in the woods by a country squire; governess Jane Eyre was engaged to her married, much older employer, Mr. Rochester; and Lady Chatterley and gamekeeper Mellors practiced buggery. If anything, the fine old books were a testament to the notion that sex was deeply relevant to the human condition and if nothing else, to timeless storytelling. Looking backward at my betters made me realize that I was shy at best, cowardly at most. Okay, I was terrified to write about sex.

I had my reasons.

During my junior year at Yale, I dated a white European graduate student who was nearly a decade older. Early on in this hazardous relationship, he took me to a friend's party. In the modest kitchen of a grad student rental, the host's wiry husband leaned against the wall, his narrow hip cocked. He looked at me then turned to ask my boyfriend my ethnicity. I was the guest of a guest, and I didn't want to embarrass anyone, but as I stared at the boxes of white wine on the Formica table, I wondered why the guy wasn't asking me. When my boyfriend answered Korean, the host's husband opened his eyes wide in delight.

"Well, all right! You know Korean girls are wild in bed."

This time, it wasn't that I was afraid of looking foolish; I was just too stupid to say anything.

When the host's husband left, my boyfriend explained that he was drunk. "Ignore it, okay?"

But I couldn't. A few minutes later, I went to the bedroom to get my coat because I wanted to leave. The boyfriend could stay if he wanted to, but I'd had enough of him and the party. When I turned around to storm off, I found that the host's husband had tailed me to the bedroom. Did I want to hook up with him? he asked. "What?" I declined and left.

Prior to the graduate student whom I dated and broke up with on a regular basis for the remainder of my college years, I'd had one serious relationship, with a boy from high school who after three years decided to go out with someone else. Before the grad student party, I had not known that Korean women were considered to be sexually wild or game enough to cheat on their boyfriends and hook up with married guys. It was 1988, and I was nineteen years old. Clearly, I needed to wise up.

Soon enough, other incidents followed, confirming that my Asian face and body were disproportionately sexualized without my say-so. When I walked down Chapel Street in New Haven, homeless white and black Vietnam veterans came up close, saying they wanted to fuck my gook cunt. The other expression used was slanty pussy. Once on a sunny spring afternoon, a homeless man touched the crotch of my baggy jeans. Ashamed and scared, I ran back to my dorm room and stayed there.

In high school, I had been an immigrant kid from Queens who took the subway on a three-hour round-trip to the Bronx each day. On weekends and summers, I worked at my parents' wholesale jewelry shop. I taught Sunday school. Most of my waking life was spent on schoolwork or reading borrowed library books. In terms of appearances, I was an unnaturally tall Korean girl with small eyes behind thick eyeglasses. My mother gave me a bob cut every two months or so by the kitchen sink. The quiet second daughter of a strict Protestant minister, my lovely mother was never told that she was pretty, and she did the same when raising her three daughters. Vanity was shameful. The body was neither repudiated nor embraced. We just didn't speak of it.

I wasn't proud of this, but I didn't know much about sex beyond my one high school boyfriend and the racy plots of hundred-year-old books. The cool girls in high school and college had elegantly knotted strings of lovers—diaries filled with notable passages. Was lovemaking beautiful and pleasurable? Sure, I believed that. Sex positive? Why not. Did I look or feel sexy? No, that would have been a stretch. So how had I become an unwitting and unqualified member of a tribe with a reputation?

I wanted some answers, so I signed up for classes in Women's Studies and Asian-American History and Literature. Alas. In print and visual media Asian women were often hookers, mail-order brides, masseuses, porn stars, dragon ladies, submissive sex slaves, and yes, cartoon characters with long black hair, red lips, and racially improbable bosoms. Asian men were sinister gangsters, inscrutable businessmen, angry nerds, and scheming eunuchs. If Asian women were oversexual, then their brothers were asexual.

The allegedly positive model minority stereotype said Asian kids were good at math, and immigrant parents were hardworking machines. My mother had been a beloved piano teacher in Seoul, and in New York, she worked behind a dusty store counter alongside my father for almost two decades without complaining. As a dutiful Korean wife, she was the portrait of the stoic, unpaid female employee in the immigrant family business model.

There was also the less spoken of yet widely pervasive and condescending notion that an Asian woman was either a victimized sex worker (your family had sold you when you were eight to the highest bidder for your virgin price), or you were a docile sexual partner of a white male loser who could never get an attractive white woman (for an obedient wife, call 1-800-jadelily). If an Asian girl dated or married a white guy, the relationship was read as suspect and imbalanced—socially, romantically, and financially. If the Asian woman married some great white male, she was despised. (See Yoko Ono.)

In my later years in college, I started to write essays, and a few were published in campus periodicals. I had written one about the sexual assault of a woman on campus. In the essay, I briefly mentioned that I had learned about the attack after returning from the aforementioned grad student boyfriend's apartment where I had spent the night. An older friend, a Korean-American divinity student, pulled me aside after he'd read it.

"You shouldn't write about the fact that you had spent the night at your boyfriend's."

"Why?"

"Because a nice Korean man won't marry you if you aren't a virgin."

"So I should lie?" My mother had never addressed virginity, yet I could not imagine lying if she asked me a direct question.

My friend looked away. "You just shouldn't tell anyone. Okay?"

He was very concerned, and although I was upset with him for a lot of reasons—insensitivity to the sexual assault of the woman; religious hypocrisy; antiquated sexism and paternalism, to name a few—I also knew he was telling me the reality for some nice Korean men and their families. That's how it was. I was contaminated, because I had lost my chastity—the most precious thing for women in most Asian countries, including the place of my birth. And what made it worse was that my boyfriend then was white. In Asian countries, there were so-called good girls and bad girls, and in 1990 New Haven, those standards applied to me nonetheless.

Throughout the twentieth century to the twenty-first, Asian governments and families in China, Japan, South Korea, the Philippines, Vietnam, Thailand, Burma, Cambodia, India, and Nepal, among others, allowed the sale of their girls for sex. Those girls who brought income to their families and nations were nevertheless permanent outcasts. My divinity school friend was trying to protect me from being called a bad woman. But I did not think of them this way. My friend thought that if I concealed my sexual history—comically brief by *Cosmo* girl standards—I might have a go at a nice Korean groom who might have me. The history of Asian prostitution and the modern advent of interracial romance had become curiously intertwined with one word: *whore*.

My husband was right. I hadn't written about sex, because I didn't want to get into it. I grew up not talking about sex, and I didn't want to begin doing it in my fiction. It wasn't just fear, it was also some perverse pride. In my writing, I'd wanted to be seen only as a serious and creative mind—an objective brain floating without a race, history, or a body. A well-furrowed brain in a mason jar of formaldehyde. I hadn't written about sex, because I was trying not to be identified with sex only.

But not writing about sex wasn't changing anything either. When I had worn my glasses, cut my hair short, donned shapeless turtleneck sweaters with loose jeans and New Balance sneakers, someone had called me an Oriental hooker anyway.

Now, I was trying to write a novel about identity (this became my first published novel). I had numerous questions about different professions in addition to race, class, and naturally, sex. There was a lot I didn't know. For another novel manuscript, I had been reading some wonderful ethnographies by cultural anthropologists, and I thought that I would model my research interviews with people who would populate my next book as if I were an anthropologist. My hero became Zora Neale Hurston—a gifted anthropologist and a remarkable novelist.

I conducted over forty interviews with men and women who shared profiles with my invented characters, spanning over a hundred hours. I would take a guy who worked in Wall Street to a fancy lunch, and ask him questions from my typed script. Where did you go to elementary school? What's the worst movie you've ever seen? Those questions were softballs, but even for the tough ones, my subjects wanted to keep talking. I might ask a married woman, "Do you like your husband?" and she would confess that she wanted to leave him.

I was the wannabe storyteller, but they were my Scheherazade. Their narratives riveted me, and I felt protective of them like an older sister who wouldn't judge. I was an unknown fiction writer with a file of rejections and a couple of published short stories in literary quarterlies you couldn't find at bookstores. But they did not mind. I listened carefully, and I promised to be confidential. The joke was that regardless of their ethnicity, they might end up being Korean in my novel anyway. The big surprise of what I learned on the field: Everyone wanted to talk about sex.

The old, dead novelists had been on the money after all. Sex and how we make love matters to everyone. My subjects wept about one-night stands, affairs gone wrong, women who left, and men who left. Those who abandoned were often as bereft. You shed your clothes; you reached for the other; you wanted to be loved, to forget, to hurt yourself, to worship, to feel something again, to control another person; and though the act passed momentarily, for good or for bad, the event was not forgettable. Sex haunted every single person—I learned this, too, from my interviews.

There was also humor and humility.

I had read in a magazine that the number one sexual fantasy for men was sex with two women. Really? When I interviewed guys who were my character studies for Harvard Business School graduates, I blurted out:

"Hmm. If you were to have a three-way, and I'm not saying you did or didn't, and really, you don't have to answer this one. I mean, so imagine if you were to have a ménage à trois, then what do you think you'd be thinking about? Like, you know, what would be going through your mind?"

All five men gave me the same answer. They'd be worried about performance and the satisfaction of both women.

"Honest?"

"Yes."

Until I read the magazine, I had never thought about three-way sex before. No one had ever asked me to join in, and it certainly wasn't my cup of chai. But all five men had thought of it before. A lot. It was obvious from the alacrity of their answers. Ménage mattered to men. Okay, then. I decided to write about it.

Then came Google—the technological revolution of our time. When I typed "Asian women" in the search engine, I got more than fourteen million hits—most of them for dubious dating sites and pornography. I may see myself as a forty-two-year-old writer, mother, wife, and former lawyer, but fourteen million hits trumped my subjective reality. The world was seeing something else when they searched for Asian women. There was a genre of pornography dedicated to Asian women, so I watched a video. In the one I saw, a middle-aged Asian woman was having sex with two men with mullets. Was I aroused? I was not. I watched for ten minutes, because that was sufficient. The characters were unattractive (I didn't realize how shallow I was), its office setting was absurd (workplace fantasies weren't doing it for me), and of course, the writing was comically bad (lousy writing could never turn me on). However, this genre was evidently popular and widespread. Not every person saw an Asian woman and thought pornography or mail-order bride, but some always would. This changed me as a writer. Could an Asian woman love a non-Asian man who fetishized her? How did pornography affect lovemaking for everyone? What did the Asian porn star think about her work? What did I think about all this?

So I wrote a scene with much of what I had seen in that film. Would anyone think the main character was me? Would anyone think that I had slept with a guy who watched porn? At this point, I had spent eleven years writing seriously yet was unable to publish a novel, so I figured no one would read this fourth manuscript anyway. When relevant, I wrote about sex, even Asian pornography and date rape, because I wanted to be honest about what was significant inside and outside my world. For most of my adult life, I had been uncomfortable with my body—my racial and sexual envelope. This time, in my pages, I thought, maybe I can talk about how it is for me, and I wrote it down.

If I had been angry about the lack of self-determination of Asian women's bodies and lives, I had been staging a feeble and arrogant protest by refusing to write about sex. Intercourse was a part of everyone's life, and it was an important part. Like it or not, it was often the defining subject for Asian women around the globe. Virgin, whore, dowry, bride price, family honor—all of these things boiled down to: did you have sex or not? By avoiding the topic, I had meant to be apolitical, but being apolitical was being political, too. As a novelist, did I want to be just political? No. I wanted pleasure, escape, and beauty in my fiction, too. And, in my invented world, I wanted sex to be authentic, and I wanted women to have real sex—uncomfortable, wonderful, awkward, delicious, humbling, empowering, and satisfying. As for the real world, one day, I wanted all us girls to call the shots about our true sex lives.

After my book was published, I gave my mother a copy. She had been a music major in college with a passion for literature. It was my mother who had guided me to read Somerset Maugham and André Gide, as well as Margaret Mitchell. She was the first artist in my life.

When she finished the book, she phoned me to tell me she liked it. I was so relieved that I didn't know what else to say. Always the tough customer, her liking it was for me the equivalent to the letter grade of an A.

Then she got real quiet.

"Mom?"

"Min Jin, do you think people have that much strange sex like the people in your book?"

"I think people have more sex and stranger sex. Sex is a part of everyone's life."

I was thirty-nine years old then, and that was my first conversation about sex with my mother.

It was a start.

My First Time, Twice

Ariel Levy

When I was fourteen years old, I decided it was time to lose my virginity. Precocity had always been my thing. As an only child, I spent most of my youth around adults, which made me sound sort of like one. By early adolescence I had become so accustomed to being told I was mature, it seemed obvious to me that this next benchmark had to be hit early in order to maintain my identity. I was curious about sex. But mostly, I had a reputation to uphold. (I was pretty much the only person interested in this reputation.)

The first—and only impressive—expression of my precociousness was when I insisted on learning to read in nursery school. I loved talking and words, and once I could write them down I was a step closer to becoming myself. The upside of being a verbal kid is that adults often think you are bright, but children have another name for such a person: nerd. As I was going through puberty (early), I saw the necessity of shifting my focus from doing things that would impress my parents and teachers, to engaging in behavior that would strike my peers as cool. I started saying *like* constantly. I smoked pot when I was twelve. I dropped acid when I was thirteen. Losing my virginity was the next logical step.

It's not that these things were necessarily fun. Well, the pot, actually, was great—unless you are reading this and *you* are twelve, in which case it was awful. But the acid was a classic bad trip, during which I thought I heard the breathing of dead people. With sex, as with drugs, my interest in the entity itself was far less potent a motivator than my fervent desire to transform myself from tiny dork into Janis Joplin. It felt like my job. I needed to do things that would make people gasp. Nobody would gasp if they heard a fifteen- or sixteen-year-old had lost her virginity. The clock was ticking.

I had a beautiful boyfriend when I was fourteen, with whom I was thoroughly infatuated. Josh had dark blue eyes and long, curly brown hair, which was (prematurely!) streaked with silver. He hung out on the steps in front of our high school with other boys who smoked cigarettes and, occasionally, joints in the bushes. Both of our sets of parents were slowly but surely separating, and both Josh and I were paradoxically desperate to assert our independence from them by mimicking the very expressions of rebellion they had taught us. We listened to Neil Young and Bob Dylan. We wore tie-dyes. We read *On the Road* and *The Prophet*. When Josh and I started going out I felt that I had been delivered from my isolation, my uncoolness, and my family. It did not occur to me that I got the ideas for my outfits from photographs of my mother taken at a time when she looked happy to be with my father.

Josh and I were unstoppable in our pursuit of 1960s-inflected accessories and experiences, but we were timid about sex. On the occasions when we found ourselves alone in bedrooms or on couches, our bravado dissipated and we became children again, unsure of what was expected of us. We did not have a lot of lust to guide us. We found each other attractive, but we were so young neither of us had ever experienced clear erotic desire. The thing I badly wanted wasn't sex, but to be rid of my virginity, the last vestige of a childhood spent trusting and respecting adults, seeking their approval. Josh, I knew, was as confused about what this entailed as I was. I never brought it up. It was all we could do to get past second base.

After Josh broke my heart, my great regret was not that I had lost my virginity to him, but that I hadn't. If I was going to be love-lorn, at least I would have liked the consolation of being able to brag that I'd had sex. So, when I was fifteen, I started going to bars with a pack of girls who went to Catholic school in Manhattan and knew how to get fake IDs. We would go to crummy dives in the East Village to drink beer, listen to awful bands, and flirt with grown men.

Once, I gave my number—or, I should say, my mother's number—to a bassist with black hair who was twenty-seven. I can't remember if he took me to dinner or to hear music, but I'm sure I had to be home by eleven, and that our conversation was stilted and humor-less. I saw him only once. I was impressed by his advanced age and how shocking it would be if I told people he was my boyfriend, but even I knew that this was not enough grist for a relationship.

I met another guy who was funny and went to film school at NYU. He was twenty-two and had a tiny apartment on Great Jones Alley, and I thought he might make a suitable boyfriend, or at least a suitable deflowerer. He was older, he'd done it before, and, I had been told, all men were dying to have sex at all times, so it would be easy enough to get him on board with my project. It was harder than I thought. He was eager to make out and grope, but to my surprise and disgust, he seemed very uneasy about engaging in ac-tual intercourse once I admitted—in the most blasé terms—that it would be my first time. It is possible this young man had located the term "statutory rape" somewhere in the back of his head. Or, per-haps his father or mother had warned him that girls get attached to their first lover—you break it you bought it, or some such. But his reluctance was no match for my romantic poetry: I told him that he didn't have to worry about me falling in love with him, and that if he wouldn't sleep with me I'd find someone else who would.

As it happened, we split the difference. He agreed to have sex with me, and to the best of my knowledge at the time, he made good on our deal. The experience was so underwhelming, so strikingly devoid of the blissful, painful, or intensely emotional sensations I'd been promised, I wondered what was wrong with everyone for imbuing intercourse with so much import. But I was thrilled to be done with it. I was fifteen years old and I had lost my virginity, ahead of everyone else's schedule, if not my own. Or so I thought.

For the following year I told anyone who asked that I was not a virgin. I'd had sex, I'd done drugs, my parents were getting a divorce—I was not popular, but you couldn't say I was prissy. Then, the summer before I turned seventeen, I went to work on the kitchen staff at a hippie sleepaway camp. Every morning I got up early to set up the hot cocoa station; every night I put the chairs on top of the tables and mopped the dining hall floor. In August, I had three days off, and one of the counselors and I got in her battered car and drove through the thick summer air from New Hampshire to Cape Cod.

Her boyfriend was in Provincetown, living out of his van, which he parked in the woods outside of town. We sat with him on Commercial Street while he played music for money and scorched ourselves brown on the beach in the afternoon sun. When night fell, we went with him to a store called Firehouse Leather to meet some of his friends who sold belts and moccasins to tourists. One of them was a tall guy named Austin with a sand-colored ponytail. I noticed he was looking at me a lot, and I didn't want him to stop. When my friends and I walked away, I turned back and caught him still staring at me, which made us both laugh.

We had a bonfire on the beach late that night. I sat in the dunes with my friend and her boyfriend and the staff of Firehouse Leather, drinking beer and watching a meteor shower flickering in the dark above us. I don't remember what we talked about, but it didn't matter. It was clear to all of us that this was special, that we would remember it, and that the night could end only one way: my friend would go back to the woods and I would walk down Commercial Street in the dawn with Austin and get into his bed.

When we had sex, it became clear to me that, in fact, I had never had sex before. What had happened on that futon on Great Jones had been a failed attempt; the young man from NYU had not completed his mission. This, now, was something else. It was uncomfortable, then pleasurable, but most of all it was different. It was different from the plodding loneliness of high school, and from the harrowing, cyclical fights with my parents that had become our routine. It wasn't boring, and it wasn't uncomplicated, and it wasn't like taking acid. It was something that was better to do than to talk about doing. It was a door to another place, another way of being that didn't have to do with language. It would take me many, many years to understand what I wanted from it, but I was so glad to know it was there.

Austin wrote me long letters that I read by the brown lake back at camp—I think I still have one in a hatbox somewhere. I saw him many times over the years, when I went up to look at the college he attended in Massachusetts, and when I went back to Provincetown for summer weekends in my twenties. We would sleep together once in a while, if we both happened to be single, and sometimes even if we didn't, until eventually we both grew up and reached the age when you stop wishing you were older and more worldly and start wishing you could be young again.

But he could have been anyone. I wasn't looking for love, though God knows I needed it. I was looking for myself. I knew so little about sex I imagined I'd experienced it years before this was true. But I knew that sex was a way to discover and communicate who you are. I don't think I was wrong about that.

Light Me Up

Margot Magowan

According to Dr. Mayfield, six weeks after the birth, Henry and I were allowed to have sex. I was so excited, I calculated the exact day, which felt at the time, to my mush brain, like doing calculus. When the moment arrived, I practically tore off his clothing. It wasn't sexual desire. I just wanted to feel like a woman instead of a cow. For a few minutes. Also, and maybe this was the same thing, I wanted to connect with Henry again, feel as if we were something more than co-caretakers of an eating, defecating mini-creature. The no-sex thing kind of stressed me out, because it was so different for us. Since we'd been together, we'd always had a lot of sex.

It was early morning. Our room was full of blue light. Ivy was asleep in the cradle next to the bed. I turned toward Henry, smiling, kissing him, pulling off his shirt and pushing off his boxers with my foot. But while that was all happening, I had a strange, disconnected feeling, like how people describe near-death experiences, as if I were floating up somewhere above my body. When we were naked, I pulled him tight against me, trying to wake my body up.

"You're ready?" he said, misunderstanding, and then went inside of me.

"Ow!" I yelled, pushing him off, my elbow jabbing into his chest. I felt as if my vagina were on fire.

"What's wrong?" he said, reaching his arm out toward the head-board, trying to regain his balance.

"It hurts. I don't know. "

Henry lay back on his side, looking down at me, one arm across my breasts. Just that was painful, his arm lying there, when I'd always adored the weight of it, of him.

"I had a C-section— why would it hurt down there?"

He shook his head.

"I thought that's why movie stars scheduled them—they don't want anything messing with their vaginas." I smiled at my reference to my *Us Weekly* obsession, which drove him crazy. But I was scared. I felt as if my body had closed up, gotten hostile. "Do you think something happened to me?" I said. "Do you think they cut a nerve?"

"No, Juliet, hypochondriac. Your body's gone through a lot."

"But Mayfield said six weeks. It's been six weeks."

He brushed my hair across my forehead with his fingers, tucking it behind my ear. "How much did it hurt?"

"So much. And it's not just that it hurt. Before that, I wasn't into it. It felt like something was happening to my body, but not to me."

He looked sad and confused.

"It's not about you," I said, touching his arm, my favorite part of his body. " It's not your fault."

"Okay," he said, sounding unsure.

"I don't know what's going on. My body doesn't feel like my body. I can't explain it."

We attempted sex a few more times over the next month, and it always felt horrible. I tried to calm myself— maybe I had a yeast infection. But I had no other symptoms.

I'd been counting on sex to make me feel better, the way it always had, my whole life, just by relaxing me, making my body feel good, just that at least. It wasn't only the pain that alarmed me. It was the lack of feeling, nothing where something used to be, coming home to a robbed house. Henry's touch seemed invasive, aggressive. Not just his dick. Wherever he touched me. My whole body felt hypersensitive. I wanted the gentlest contact. The kind of feather touch I thought I hated, that tickled me and made my skin crawl. Usually, I liked to be pressed hard or grabbed tight. But now I craved cuddling, no dirty sex talk, but a paternal or maybe a maternal kind of love.

There were other differences I noticed in myself. Sex, or even just blatant sexuality, on TV disgusted me—watching reality shows' horny drunks or all those women shaking their asses in videos. Previously, even when I didn't like something that was on, I often got sucked in, fascinated, curious, analyzing, trying to figure it all out. Now it was just gross.

If I came across a porn channel while flipping through the remote, I actually got nauseated. My reaction to it was so extreme, so physical, I worried I might team up with an army of right-wing suburban housewives from the Bible belt to launch an antiporn crusade.

Sex was becoming something I just didn't get, like looking at food after you've had a big meal and you can't imagine ever being hungry again. I didn't pick up sexual innuendos or imagery. Once, while Ivy was sleeping, and I was looking at a magazine, I saw a photo of a woman licking an ice cream and I got my queasy, porno reaction. When I saw her giant tongue on a red, wet Popsicle and made the obvious sexual connection, I realized I hadn't been aware of that kind of stuff for a long time.

That was weird, because I'd made a whole career out of picking all that up, highlighting semidisguised, accepted, ubiquitous misogyny. I was an assistant professor of cultural studies at UC Berkeley, and one of my skills, exploited in both my dissertation and my book (if I ever finished it) was my ability to spot phallic symbols and "vaginal" ones too. I even won kudos from my dissertation panel for pointing out that the latter had never been assigned a literary term. The sexual semiotics were so obvious to me, I didn't understand how people could miss them. The very first time I saw the Joe Camel ad, when I was twelve, I couldn't believe they'd created a cartoon face out of a penis and two fat, droopy testicles. Of course, a lot of people caught on eventually, but when they finally banned that pervy camel, they said it was because he was an animated character, appealing to kids. None of those congressmen seemed bothered that his face was a penis.

Having no sexual desire anymore confused me about Henry. I didn't know what he was for. I knew that sounded awful. It was awful. I couldn't believe I was thinking such mean, horrible thoughts—a new mom. But it wasn't just that he couldn't give me orgasms. He couldn't breast-feed either. He didn't make much money. He'd forget to pick up diapers. He didn't buy the vibrating chair or the baby monitor, or any of that endless baby paraphernalia you need, until I asked him to about a hundred times. He'd forget to pay his cell phone bill, which was huge, never dealing with signing up for a cheaper plan, so my calls would go straight to voice mail. I saw his flaws everywhere, the way I used to see phallic symbols. Maybe I'd made a horrible mistake getting into this marriage thing. How had my life changed so fast anyway? Was it lust that got me here? A broken condom?

The first time I saw Henry, about two years prior, I wandered into his lamp store in the Mission. He made these crazy, beautiful lamps, and he was so intense about them, bent over them with a million tools that looked exactly the same to me, but later, he explained, were all slightly different; it's all about how they're angled. I'd never been attracted to a blond guy before, but it was his gray eyes that hooked me, the furrow between them shaped like a backward *K*. I wanted him to study me the way he did those lamps, with that kind of focused attention, as if I were that fascinating and complicated, unusual and beautiful; make him figure out how to light me up.

He didn't even notice me when I walked into his store, and I have to admit, that was part of the initial attraction. Bored in bars from New York City to Austin, I'd make seduction a game: could I make the guy totally absorbed in something else become absorbed in me? Could I make him have sex with me again and again and be late for work? Miss work altogether? Miss a plane?

"This is so pretty," I said, pointing to the lampshade Henry was working on. He was weaving together copper strands in loose, wiry braids over an exposed yellow bulb, all of which cast sharp, black shadows across the walls like giant spiderwebs. "How much is it?"

"It's not finished yet," he said, twisting some copper so it hooked over the wrought-iron, pentagon-shaped shade.

"Isn't it almost done though?" I said. "I could wait."

He looked over at me, shook his hair out of his face, and smiled.

At some point, watching him all hunched over, I said something like, "Are you OK? Don't you want to sit up?" I walked over to him. "That position looks so uncomfortable. Let me rub your head for a while." I reached out and touched his neck and then his hair. I gave him the most incredible neck/head/hair massage, intended to relax and arouse him all at once. I was successful.

I hit on Henry that day, it's true. But it was Henry who fell in love first, who came to adore me and told me so all the time, who wanted to be exclusive just three weeks later and then wanted to marry me. By the time he officially proposed with his grandmother's ring, a daisy chain of pavé and yellow diamonds, seven months later, I was in love with him too.

Marriage had never been in my life plan or dream or whatever. Nor had kids. My parents had a bitter divorce, I loved my work, and I wasn't into the whole commitment thing. But I was so infatuated with

Henry that I'd started to wonder what it would be like to make a baby with him. He came from a huge Catholic family; he loved kids, and kids loved him back. So I told him I'd think it over. Then the condom broke. He agreed to get married in Vegas, after the morning sickness had passed, just him and me. That plan won me over.

For our honeymoon, my mom gave us a gift certificate for two nights at a five-star hotel in Santa Barbara. But we decided to save the trip for when I wasn't pregnant and the baby was old enough to leave with a sitter. I wanted to go when I could feel sexy in my bikini and drink margaritas by the pool, worry free.

But now, six months after my wedding, up at 3:00 A.M. nursing Ivy, I was starting to obsess about that hotel. A place like that could be just what Henry and I needed, a change of scene and some real romance. How could you not have great sex at a place like that? I got up and went to my desk, digging out the brochure. My mouth dropped open as I looked at the glossy photos, fantasizing about the clean towels, the room service, and the giant TV. The resort seemed to offer everything I craved. I was breast-feeding 24/7, why not do it with an ocean view? When Henry woke up the next day, I told him I wanted to go as soon as possible, convincing him it would be good for us.

When we arrived, the concierge gave us flutes of champagne and then we got a ride on a golf cart to our room. The suite had billowing curtains opening onto a balcony overlooking the ocean. There was a giant bed with a white comforter on a shiny, blue tile floor, like a puffy cloud in a perfect sky. There was another room with panoramic windows, a huge fruit bowl on a glass coffee table, and a crib for Ivy. While she slept there, we used the two-headed shower and then got in the sunken tub together. Henry stretched out across the whole bath, his arms and legs spilling over the sides like an overgrown plant.

We put on bathrobes and opened the doors to the patio so we could look out at the sea right from the bed. I started playing with his penis. When it got hard, he pulled me on top of him so his mouth was in between my legs and I was facing the headboard. That position annoyed me. It was the only way he ever went down on me. I couldn't concentrate on coming, because I was so worried I'd smother him. He always told me it was okay, he had been a competitive swimmer and could hold his breath. I knew that was part of the turn-on, too, being smothered by pussy and all, and I was all for that every now and then, especially after years of choking on cock. But now, my breasts dribbling milk, him gasping for air, it just didn't feel sexy. I knew that after fifteen minutes of it, Henry would get pissed I wasn't coming. Then he would ask what was wrong with me. We were headed to a bad place, so instead of trying to struggle through, I aborted, getting up and off of him. It was the first time I'd ever stopped oral sex in the middle like that.

"What's going on?" he asked.

"Nothing, I'm just not into this right now."

"What?"

"I don't feel like having sex."

"Why? Did I do something wrong?"

I sighed. He was going to make me say it. "I hate that position. It's the only way you go down on me. Once in a while it's okay, but that's the only way you do it."

Henry got up, pulled on his terry cloth bathrobe, and stomped out onto the balcony. I couldn't believe he was acting like such a baby. I got up and went out after him, naked, saying, "This is my honeymoon! It's supposed to be romantic. Why can't you just go down on me like a normal person?"

"It sounds like you don't like having sex with me," he said.

"I just don't like how you're so passive. I don't like how I always have to initiate sex. I don't like how I'm always sucking your dick and doing everything you want sexually, except anal sex and I even do that, and you never go down on me unless it's a special occasion and then you want me to sit on your face!"

"It sounds like you have a lot of problems with me," he said, looking as furious and mean as he could in his fuzzy robe.

"I wish I liked it," I said. "I hate how you make me feel like a prude or like there's something wrong with me. I don't get why you don't put some effort into having sex with me the way I like it."

"You're crazy if you don't think I put effort into pleasing you. All I do is try to please you."

"I Googled face-sitting," I said.

"You *what*?"

"The last time. I was just trying to figure stuff out. I typed that in. I didn't even know it was a word. I thought I made it up."

"Jesus."

"Hundreds of sites came up. Mostly dominatrix ones. Women stabbing shoes into men's faces. I know you're not into that, so it just confirmed for me—it's the most passive way for you to go down on me."

"You're insane."

"But can you just tell me why you don't try to figure out what I like? Is it that you're too good-looking? You never had to try that hard? God, I just had a baby, I'm breast-feeding all night long! And then you want me to sit on your face!"

"Oh my God," he said, "I want a lactating woman to sit on my face? That *is* fucked up." He smiled. "That wasn't exactly my fantasy growing up."

He made me laugh. I couldn't help it. I stood there on the patio, naked and laughing.

That night we ordered room service and watched a Lauren Bacall movie on our TV. There were a few candles in the room, and we lit them all, leaving the doors open all night and listening to the sea.

In the morning Henry woke up with a hard-on and wanted sex again, but I was too sleepy, so he masturbated on my ass. Henry loved my ass. He said it was my fault, that I made him act that way, all sex crazy about my ass. It took him a long time to come, maybe because I wasn't paying attention to him at all. He never used lubricant, he thought it was cold and slimy, but he rubbed so hard and long that when he was done, there was a sore on his dick. It hurt him so badly, he wouldn't let me touch him for days.

Our sex life pretty much ground to a halt after that weekend, though there were a few more lame attempts. Some nights, when tiny Ivy was asleep, I'd be the one to go find Henry. Seek him out while he'd was working on a lamp downstairs to see if that former turn-on would do it for me now. I started kissing him. I was going to seduce him again, fuck my way back to my true identity. I'd sit on his lap, wrap my legs around him. But his mouth seemed so wet, his tongue heavy and gross, reminding me of the Popsicle ad that had turned my stomach. He reached out to hold me closer to him, his fingers pressing hard into my arm, which hurt. I pushed him off of me. "What's going on?" he said, seeming frustrated and confused and angry with me too.

"I don't know."

"If you don't want to have sex, fine. But this starting-stopping drives me crazy."

"I want to and then I don't." I started to cry. "I don't know what's wrong with me."

"It's okay," he said, stroking my hair. "That's what lionesses do during sex, you know—they throw the lion off of them."

"I feel defective," I said. "Imagine if all of a sudden you were impotent."

He nodded. "That would be hard. I mean difficult."

I smiled, in spite of myself.

"Let's just try to be patient," he said.

"But how? What are you doing? Are you masturbating? In the shower or something?"

"Please stop worrying so much," he said. "This will pass."

Part of what was so mystifying to both of us about my alien body was that it looked just like my body. I'd lost all the baby weight immediately, just like my star friends in *Us Weekly* who waxed poetic, in cover story after cover story, about their victorious postbaby weight losses. Yet they had nothing at all to share about any lack of sex drive, postpartum, with their Sexiest Man Alive husbands.

In fact, no one had much to say about it. I read over all my pregnancy books, searching for information. In the *Girlfriend's Guide to Pregnancy,* which was supposed to be so candid and frank, there was this glib advice: "inebriate and lubricate." Of course, now I knew what that meant. But the pregnancy expert only gave some lame, vague explanation for those recommended accoutrements, like feeling fat or unattractive.

Nothing I read described my problem, exactly. The books referred to exhaustion, or physical healing of vaginal tears. There was nothing about disliking his touch or disliking him. There was quite a lot of information about postpartum depression. That seemed closer to how I felt than anything I read about sex. But I didn't really fit that either. I wasn't depressed about my baby. I thanked God for my baby, otherwise I really would've felt as if I took a wrong turn. I wasn't indifferent about Ivy or having any thoughts about hurting her or feeling like I couldn't care for her.

When my friend Sheila called me, I finally told her what was going on with Henry and me. Just a few years ago, confiding in her would've been no big deal. But I'd resisted for a couple of reasons. Sheila wanted a baby so badly, I felt like I couldn't complain to her about any negative side effects of the whole birth miracle. She had a miscarriage right around the time I got pregnant.

Another reason I avoided talking to Sheila was because of something she'd said that haunted me. She had told me once, crying, that her husband, Stephen, didn't seem to care whether or not they had kids. That shocked me, because I knew Sheila was desperate to be a mom. When I asked her why she had never told me about how Stephen felt, she rolled her eyes and said: *Married people don't talk about their relationships.*

It wasn't just that my best friend said that to me. Now I felt it. To speak about my unhappiness or confusion seemed disloyal, a betrayal of Henry. It also scared me, because I needed him. But then I wondered: Was never speaking of it really so great for the relationship? That idea reminded me of not swearing in front of a lady or being careful not to upset an old man on the verge of a heart attack; it implied my marriage was too fragile to withstand *words.* So I talked.

"You weren't into it," Sheila said. "What's the big deal? Jesus, calm down. It's not the end of the world. Haven't you ever had bad sex before?"

"No," I said. "Not like that. I mean, I've been with inept guys. I've had frustrated moments. And I've been not satisfied."

"Well . . ."

"But this is different. This isn't like not getting something I want. It's not *wanting.*"

"Welcome to married life."

"Are you serious? Don't joke about this."

"Look, I don't know how babies factor in. It probably takes a while to get your sex drive back. Call Alicia or Jennifer. Ask them."

Alicia or Jennifer would have been good choices if my friends still talked about their relationships. Like me, they'd met their husbands and got pregnant quickly. I actually knew a lot of women my age who'd done that, maternity wedding dresses and all. Vera Wang should've designed a line just for my slutty generation of thirty-something women, careless brides who got knocked up and tied the knot like it was something that was meant to go together in one sitting, a well-balanced meal, meat and potatoes. Of those paired events, having a baby was supposed to be the big deal, the life-altering event. Getting married wasn't really supposed to *change* anything.

"I can't just call people up and ask if their vaginas hurt. You basically said that yourself. Wives don't talk."

"Listen, Juliet, don't make such a big deal out of this. Just fake it, act like you're having a good time."

"What?"

"Just fake it. Everyone's happier that way. Trust me."

I felt so separate from her; she didn't get me at all. It was like when I was in labor and felt all alone.

"They're lots of things you can do," Sheila went on. "Try fantasizing about someone else. It's no big deal."

"But I got married because I was in love with Henry. Not to fake orgasms."

"Oh, come on Pollyanna. Lust fades. Everyone knows that. Baby or no baby."

"But I don't believe lust has to fade. I think it's more complicated than that. I don't think that's a given."

"Okay, so you guys are the exception," Sheila said. "I don't want to be a downer. Call your doctor about the pain."

I called the advice nurse at Mayfield's office. "Sex hurts."

"It's hormones," she said. "Thinned vaginal walls. That will get better when you stop breast-feeding. Use lubricant."

So I went out to buy a couple of kinds. I went to a sex store called Good Vibrations in the same neighborhood where Henry worked. I'd been there a few times before, but it all repulsed me now, the purple dildos stacked on counters and black leather harnesses and chains hanging off the walls. It occurred to me that maybe my sex disgust was a form of birth control, making sure you spaced babies apart in a healthy way. I thought I'd even heard something like that before, though attributed to not menstruating while breast-feeding. But if that were true, it seemed so harsh of God. And limited, linear thinking, confining sex to reproduction. I'd just given birth after ten months of pregnancy. Didn't I deserve an orgasm?

So I bought three different kinds and even picked up some free samples. But Henry hated lubricant. When he groaned at the sight of my purchases, I thought back to the sore on his dick and felt hopeless. He finally gave in, but I felt like a controlling, nagging wife when I wanted to be a sex goddess.

And the thing is, when he did use the lubricant, it still didn't feel good. Nothing felt good. I stared to wonder if I should fake orgasms like Sheila had said, just to get it over with. But that idea felt so bad and against everything I believed in. Lying about something so intimate was unthinkable. Except that I *had* thought it. And even if I didn't do it, I understood doing it. That was new.

But if it were true that great sex was something you grew out of, not into, I honestly couldn't believe no one had warned me. Or maybe the whole world had, with all those impersonal, ubiquitous clichés like "infatuation fades." But hadn't we also been sold true love? Didn't that include passion? And if it didn't, why had no friend sat me down and let me in on all this before I'd gone and married my sexy husband whom I had planned on fucking and maybe supporting for the rest of my life?

In an attempt to get my mind off my troubled sex life and disconnected marriage, I often took long walks or focused on potentially distracting and mundane tasks like paying bills. Henry still hadn't made it to the AT&T wireless place to get a cheaper plan, so I decided to combine distractions: go for a walk with Ivy and get a new plan.

There was no line in front of the Asian guy with spiky hair who sat behind the counter. He had a cell phone in parts laid out in front of him, and his furrowed brow and row of tools made me think of the first time I met Henry.

"I'm late on my bill," I said, sitting down in the swivel chair across from him, "which is really high. Can you take a look at the charges? Maybe I could get on another plan."

"How high is it?"

"It was over three hundred dollars last month."

He looked at me, tilting his head. "That's high."

"It's two phones, my husband's and mine. I could've missed a payment, too."

"Still," he said, shaking his head, spinning around in his own chair to face his computer. "Have you been buying anything on it?"

"Buying anything?" I repeated.

"You can get stuff off the Web and charge your phone," he said.

"I didn't even know that," I said, thinking—so, that's how Henry bought the vibrating chair. The baby monitor. All that stuff I was so grateful he finally purchased. "Maybe my husband . . ."

"You have no extra charges on your bill." He shrugged. "What's your husband's number?"

I rested my elbows on the counter, looking at the tiny, dissected phone parts while he tapped keys.

"There's something on your husband's account," he said. He turned the screen to me.

I saw rows and rows of the same five-digit sequence and across from each of those $9.99 going down his screen into infinity. "What is that?" I said. "I don't understand."

He pointed to a third column. "It says mobile dating."

I leaned close to the screen, shielding my eyes, as if it were a sunny day; I was so near that my pinky was touching the computer, making a color swirl. "Mobile dating," I read. "Oh my God. Mobile dating!" My mouth felt sticky when I tried to speak again. "Phone sex? Is this phone sex?"

"I don't really know," he said. "It says 'dating.' It looks like he's been using a dating service."

"A dating service? Oh my God." I rested my head in my hands, so I was looking down at Ivy, who was half awake in her sling. I ran my finger down the curve of her cheek, checking the rolls in her neck, the places where milk and dirt sometimes collected in gray pellets. Ivy looked back at me, blinking patiently. Her eyes were still that newborn navy blue color but getting lighter all the time. I just sat there, looking down at her, my eyes fixed on hers.

Finally the guy said to me, "I can look up that service for you if you'd like. Maybe we can figure out what it is."

"Would you mind?" I said, disappointed that in the silence he hadn't just disappeared, along with his computer and all the information it contained. "That would be really helpful. Thank you."

"Okay, sure." He typed, paused, typed. "Yeah—it looks like a dating service." He pointed to the screen that was still facing me. There was an image of a girl wearing a black beret and black tank top, red lipstick, smiling. She was holding a cell phone. Next to her the words, which he read out loud, "Meet local singles in your town." Then a new photo came on the screen, a girl lying down, also in a tank top, that one pink, her arms stretched out in front of her, in her hands a white cell phone. "Real singles, just a phone call away."

"Oh my God," I said again.

"I'm sorry," he said. "Do you want me to print out the bill?"

"Can you do that? Could you check the other months?"

"It's on last month's too," he said. "I already checked. I'll look at April." After a minute he said, "April too. We only keep records three months back."

He printed it all for me, and when I left the store, my fingers were shaking so much that I could barely dial Henry's number on the stupid, fucking cell phone. "I need to talk to you. Can you meet me at Noah's on Chestnut Street?"

"What's up?" he said.

"I'll wait for twenty minutes. After that, I'm leaving."

"Leaving? What do you mean leaving?" he said.

I turned the phone off and went across the street into Noah's. I sat on the patio at a wrought-iron table in the cold and the fog, hugging warm and sleeping Ivy to me. I kept thinking how stupid I was and how every woman probably thinks the same thing. I never thought he would be with someone else. I had no fucking idea. How could I miss something like this? At least now things were clear. Get away from this loser, idiot, lamp maker. Lamp maker, seriously. He was hot, but I married him? I had a baby with him?

I recognized him by his walk, which was more of a lope, his torso hanging back, and his legs striding ahead, like an R. Crumb cartoon. I knew he could see my face even from the sidewalk, through two sets of glass doors, because he had eagle eyes. He was always pointing out things to me I never would have seen or noticed, like the dot of a hawk in the sky or a silver rectangle across the bay that was the hospital where he was born. And it wasn't just his vision. All his senses were heightened. He heard things and smelled things seconds before I did. And watching him walk through Noah's, past the line of people ordering their lunch, to get to me, I couldn't breathe, because somehow I knew I loved him. Still. I knew it all again, just like that.

He sat down next to me and looked at the bill, three sheets of white paper that I'd laid out on the table. The phone numbers were circled, "mobile dating" underlined several times. He looked across the patio, his arms crossed on his chest. Then he wove his fingers together, pressed them outward so his knuckles cracked, crossed his arms again. "I was masturbating," he said.

"You're such a fucking liar."

"You didn't want to have sex with me," he said.

"So this is why you were so calm about our shitty sex life." I turned to him, my face so close to his that I could see the light stubble on his cheek. "Now I get it. Just be patient—ha!"

"You seemed like you lost all desire for me."

"Do you realize I just had a fucking baby? Something happened to my body!"

"That's why I didn't want to bother you," he said.

"I tried to talk to you about it. Oh my God." I hit my elbow hard onto the table, my funny bone throbbing. I was grateful for the physical pain, the jolt of it helping me to stay angry, which was better than experiencing how scared I was. I could feel sadness, just below the skin of my face, a body under water, about to surface.

"I felt like you wanted nothing to do with me. Except to feel better about yourself."

"How do you think I felt? You did nothing to inspire sexual feelings in me. You came to me with your sexual needs but there was no romance. I asked you about masturbating and you didn't say anything!"

"I was ashamed."

"Ashamed of what exactly? Were you with someone else?"

"No."

"You weren't with anyone else? I don't believe you. I don't believe you were 'just masturbating' or whatever. How do I know what the fuck you were doing? Why would you go to a *dating* service to masturbate? Even the AT&T wireless guy didn't think it was just phone sex."

"The AT&T wireless guy?" he said.

"He looked it up for me on the Internet."

"I wasn't trying to meet anyone."

"Then why *that* service?"

"Because it was free."

"Because it was *free*? Oh my God. Are you insane? Do you see this bill?" I picked up the papers and held them right in front of his face. "Hundreds of dollars! I was complaining to you about this bill for weeks!" I stood up.

"I saw an ad in *SF Weekly*. It said the first call was free."

"Look how many calls you made, asshole," I said.

"You don't understand," he said. "Each call wasn't . . ." He trailed off.

"What?"

"I wasn't talking to anyone."

"Right, you were having an affair."

"No."

"Fuck you, Henry." I got up out of my chair, my arm underneath the sling, keeping Ivy still.

"Wait," he said, grabbing my arm. "Let me explain. Please."

I stood there, looking through the glass doors, through the restaurant, out onto the street where I could see people walking.

"It was a message exchange. People record messages, and I listened to them. There was no connection."

"What did the messages say?"

"Sexual things, stupid things. Like 'I just got out of the shower, I'm horny.'"

"What did your messages say?"

"My messages?" he sounded surprised. "I didn't record any. Well, I recorded one. You have to record one to do it."

"What did it say?"

He was quiet.

"Tell me."

"This is Michael. I'm six one. I have gray eyes."

"Oh God. That's so real. That makes me feel sick."

"I'm sorry, Juliet. I felt so rejected by you. I felt like you didn't want me. You seemed so angry and so unsatisfied."

"I tried to talk to you about how I felt. I needed you to be there for me. But you were never there for me and this whole thing is a lie. I'll never be able to trust you again."

I walked out of Noah's without looking back, pressing bundled

Ivy close against me, moving faster and faster until I was practically running. The cold fog felt so good on my burning face. I went straight to Sheila's house. I didn't call her to let her know I was coming, because I couldn't bring myself to turn on my cell phone.

Sheila opened her door, looking beautiful as always, in a white turtleneck and white pants. I couldn't remember the last time I wore white. "Hey, this is a nice surprise," she said. And then, "What's wrong?"

I collapsed against her, bawling like a child, which woke Ivy up and made her cry too.

Sheila put her arms around me, holding me, all of us staying in her doorway until I pushed her away to take a deep breath, wiping my nose on my sleeve.

"Come get a Kleenex," she said, taking Ivy from me.

"I am a Kleenex," I said. "I'm covered in spit-up and snot. It makes no difference. Really."

Sheila smiled and reached out to touch Ivy's cheek. "Hey, precious," she said. Keeping her arm around me, she guided us inside. "I'll make you some tea."

She handed Ivy down to me as I sat on her white couch and looked through her giant rectangular window at the two bridges, the Golden Gate on one side and the Bay Bridge on the other, Alcatraz Island in the middle, the view from Pacific Heights that everyone in San Francisco wanted. I could hear Sheila moving things around in her kitchen.

"My cell phone bill has been really high," I said, unclipping my bra so I could nurse Ivy. "So I went to the wireless place, and it turns out . . ." I cupped my hand under Ivy's tiny, bald head, marveling at how she curved perfectly into my palm. "It turns out Henry's been calling a mobile dating service. Hundreds of dollars of calls. Over months. As far back as the records go."

Sheila came out of the kitchen, holding a metallic purple teakettle, the kind that makes a two-toned harmonica sound instead of a whistle. "Oh God, Juliet." She stood in front of me, the kettle in midair. "Was he having sex with these women?"

"He told me he was masturbating. No face-to-face encounters with anyone. He said he didn't want to meet anybody. It's some kind of message exchange."

"What?"

"He told me, I don't know if it's true, but he told me he listened to messages."

"That's not such a big deal," Sheila said. "Everybody masturbates."

I was having a déjà vu of our earlier conversation, about faking orgasms and other lies Sheila had supported *for the sake of the relationship*. How stupid and smug I'd been then, thinking Henry and I were so honest, so open with each other, above all that.

"But he never told me about it."

"He was probably ashamed."

"That's exactly what he said." I twisted my hair around in my hand. "But ashamed of what?"

"Phone sex is OK as long as it's not one of those, you know, meet real people places."

"That's exactly what it was," I said.

Sheila put the teakettle down on the ottoman. She plucked a pink Kleenex from the box next to it, handing it to me. I took it from her and blew my nose, then pulled a folded square of paper from my diaper bag, holding it toward her. "Go look up mobile dating and this number on your computer. You'll see what I saw."

She unfolded the bill, and Ivy turned toward her, because she loved the sound of paper.

"This doesn't say anything," Sheila said, squinting at the numbers. "Except that he was being compulsive with the calls. He was calling a lot. Look, every day that week."

"Yeah, I thought he had a low sex drive. Ha!"

She went across the room, sat down, and typed. "Okay, it's real women, which is bad," she said, looking at me over the monitor. "But if he wasn't a member, it doesn't look like he could do much. According to these charges, nine dollars and ninety-nine cents a pop, it doesn't look like he was a member. Where's he now?" she asked.

I reached in the diaper bag again, turned my phone back on, and right then it rang. I had twelve missed calls from him. I turned it off again. "Can I lie down with Ivy? I just feel like going to sleep."

She put me in her guest room with its cream-colored comforter and silky pillows. I changed Ivy's diaper and cuddled next to her warm little body. I fell asleep right away, because crying a lot exhausts me; just like a little kid, I pass out. When I woke up, it was dark. I pushed Ivy to the middle of the bed, put a blanket over her lower half, and went into the living room.

"Henry called here," she said. "That's probably what woke you. I told him you were sleeping. He said he was coming by."

"Please don't let him in."

About fifteen minutes later, the doorbell rang. Sheila changed the channel to *Entertainment Tonight,* then CNN. The bell rang a couple more times. Then Sheila's phone. It rang again.

Sheila turned to me. "This can't go on. I've got to get it. This is ridiculous." She reached up behind her, over the back of the couch, grabbing the phone from the table. "Henry, if you don't go away, I'm going to call the police." She listened and then hung up. "He says he loves you and he's sorry."

I shrugged.

"He says he won't call or ring the doorbell, but he'll wait outside my house until you talk to him."

"Fuck him," I said.

"He said he'll wait all night."

Ivy started crying, and I went in the guest room to get her. I brought her to the couch and nursed her. Sheila opened some wine, but I didn't feel like any. About an hour later, she made pasta, but neither of us ate it. After a while, she left out a plate for Stephen on the dining room table, and we all went to bed.

I stayed with Sheila for four days before I saw Henry again. Sometimes, I tried hard to see things from his point of view. I realized I hadn't really done that at all, the whole time. I didn't think he deserved that effort, since I'd gone through so much with the pregnancy, birth, breast-feeding, etcetera. But I saw how I'd mostly used sex with him just to feel okay about myself. Maybe I'd always used sex for that.

Sheila said she'd watch Ivy when I went to meet him. She was so excited to have the baby all to herself, I ended up leaving her place twenty minutes early. When I got home, I went upstairs to wash my face. Henry's shirt was on the floor, and I picked it up to throw it in the laundry basket. Then I just sat with it on the bed until he came home.

"Hey," he said. "Nice to see you." He sat down next to me and took my hand. "Juliet, I love you. I've missed you. I'm sorry about all this. I understand what you must be feeling."

"I don't feel like you understand," I said. "If I did this to you, you'd leave me." I started to cry. "I feel so betrayed and lied to."

"I don't feel like I betrayed you. I just felt like you didn't want me."

"So that made you go off with another person?"

"There was no other person. It was a fantasy world."

"Why can't you explore your fantasies with me?"

"I want to, but you're so in your head, Juliet. Every second. Everything has to be analyzed and processed. I just wanted to fuck you. Look"—he took my hands—"you're my wife. I don't want my wife saying things to me like why can't I have 'normal' sex."

"I asked you why you couldn't go down on me like a normal person! I felt ugly!" I took a breath and said, "I'm sorry I ever said that."

"You say shit like that to me all the time. It hurts my feelings. Maybe I thought you were incredibly sexy right then."

"I didn't feel sexy."

"But you were sexy, and you're sexy right now."

I looked at his gray eyes looking back into me, the darker gray outline around his iris, his furrowed brow.

"It was nice walking in the house and seeing you here."

He kept looking at me, studying me, all his attention on me. Time slowed, each of his movements a separated frame of an old film.

"I always had a fantasy of walking in on a girl. A girl that looks just like you. She doesn't know I'm there. Skirt hiked up. Silky panties. She's touching herself. By the time you notice me, you're too horny to stop. "

I couldn't help smiling. "Makes me wonder where this is leading."

"Let me rub your head for a while." He undid my hair from my ponytail, dropping the elastic on the floor, pushing his fingers down past my ear to my neck. "I'm really happy you're home."

Herman and Margot

Karen Abbott

How could Herman not notice Margot? Look at her: silver hair sculpted and sprayed into miniature mountain peaks, lowered lids flashing bolts of blue liner, origami skin freshly powdered and brightly rouged. Jeweled rings blink from fingers and a gold bracelet slinks around a tapered ankle. White linen slacks hide a pair of dancer's legs that kicked across every stage in the Catskills. Hot pink blazer and orthopedic sandals—not shoes—stacking enough heel to make a difference. She fairly glides in her walker. She's lived eighty-seven years, and nothing suggests she couldn't handle eighty-seven more.

He spots her in the lobby of Kittay House, a senior living community in the Bronx, and she looks like she needs him. Everyone at Kittay House has needed Herman at one time or another: to serve as president and treasurer of the board; to teach gin rummy; to make intricate, customized birthday and bar mitzvah and sympathy cards; to offer nips of grape wine from the Sprite bottle he keeps stashed in his closet. As the unofficial patriarch of the place, it would be rude and neglectful of him not to approach this fine lady and find out exactly what she wants, and so he aims his walker in her direction.

"How do you go about ordering an air conditioner?" she asks.

"I'll do it for you," he says, and it is settled.

In the beginning they take things slowly, reveling in the irony of teasing time when they have so little of it left. Margot invites him up to her apartment to watch *Dancing with the Stars*. They sit side by side in matching recliners, legs kicked up, overstuffed arms close enough to touch. He's gorgeous, by far the best man she's seen here, clean-cut in his polo shirt and black trousers and spotless white sneakers. Herman, too, looks young for his age—ninety-two—and no one doubts him when he boasts he can easily pass for eighty. They discover they share a birthday, March 13. How clever of fate to pair them now, near the end, with someone who began from the same place, a cosmic alignment that both comforts and provokes. They revel in their similar virtues—both are spirited, funny, adventurous—and neither recognizes that they also possess the same faults. She obstinately insists that he is too opinionated; his strong opinion is that she's too obstinate. Being with each other is like de facto introspection, soul searching without either angst or epiphany. It allows them to explore the nature of desire, at any age, and what a person is obliged to do with it.

One day Herman presents Margot with a bottle of cologne and waits for her reaction, his wide smile pushing his brows into a furry white *V. I have to retrain him,* she thinks and decides to tell him the truth. "You don't give me cheap cologne," she says, "something you buy over the counter for three or four dollars. A little bottle of *perfume* costs fifty dollars. It has to be name brand, Estée Lauder. I won't use that junk." He has an irritating habit of speaking for her, and interrupting her, and bringing her food—cakes and cookies and plates of cheese—when he knows damn well she wants to lose ten pounds. He calls her—*all* women, really—"dame" and "pussycat." Worse, his romantic technique lacks preamble and subtlety. No caressing of her arm, no whispering in her ear the words she's heard all her life: You're the prettiest girl in the room. It seems he has fourteen hands, clutching her arm and grabbing at her neck, and when he kisses her his mouth lands heavy on hers, as if it dropped from stories above. She calls him The Wolf.

Herman won't hear any of it. The thing is, even if he were a young man, he wouldn't marry Margot. He takes her to City Island for dinner, and all she does is complain they never go anywhere else. During a trip to Las Vegas he buys her a necklace from a shop at Caesar's Palace. "I don't like it," she says, her lips (*but God, those lips!*) sputtering in disgust. "If you gave me a hundred dollars I wouldn't wear it." She is difficult and contrary. She has her own ideas. She won't listen to him or deviate from her structured but nonsensical path. Not wife material, but she's the kind of dame he'd "have a fling with," that's for sure, and as he pays more visits to apartment 12H he dares himself to go further and further, both old enough to know better and too old to care.

Margot reminds herself that comparisons do no good, that, at her age, the now never quite equals the then. Yet she can't help but think of Bill, her first and only husband. They met in 1938, the winter after she turned twenty, when she and a girlfriend took a train from Manhattan to the Bronx for a party. Her girlfriend whirled off into the crowd, and Margot noticed a tall, thin man with a glorious head of hair, thick and black as her own. He sat alone on a piano stool, taking up only half, as if he'd been expecting her. She approached him, bold and brazen, and said, "Is this other half being occupied?" and sat down before he had time to answer.

They eloped two years later, on New Year's Eve. She wore a sleek black satin dress embroidered with white gardenias, and Bill took her on a honeymoon to Lakewood, New Jersey. They checked into a motel, the first one Margot had ever been inside, and rented a room. A heater cackled and hissed from one corner and a jukebox loomed in the other. Bill told her she deserved romantic music and dropped a quarter in the slot; somehow, Bill's selection was thwarted in favor of "Alexander's Ragtime Band." They laughed and he carried her to the bed, lowering her by inches, with excruciating care. All night long the heater belched a sooty gray mist that blackened the sheets and coated their bodies, and they didn't notice till morning. *My God,* Margot thought, *he's killing me,* and tucked herself tight and safe inside the pain until she found the sweet, secret pleasure around its edges.

She holed up in that spot Bill made especially for her for fifty-six long years. Every night, as soon as the kids were put to bed, he pulled her back there. When her sister visited and slept in their bed because they had no place else to offer her, Bill didn't care; he reached for Margot anyway, laughed when she closed her mouth against his kisses and returned his hands to his sides. Toward the end, when he smoked nearly all of his insides away, he still had the strength to want her. She'll never forget, helping him up the stairs after surgery, not five minutes home from the hospital, and there Bill was, yanking at her skirt and pulling at her buttons. "He was quite a lover," she says, and she never had anyone to compare him to, until now, until Herman.

It's funny, Herman thinks, how Margot is a precise amalgamation of his two wives. The first, Yetta, was stunning, but ornery and temperamental. He had to see the movies she wanted to see, eat only at her chosen restaurants. She refused to help him with his department store in the Bronx, where he worked ten hours a day, seven days a week. He realized, during the thirty-five years of his marriage, that he didn't exactly hate her, but he certainly didn't like her. What he did was grow used to her, tolerate her for the sake of their three children. When he retired in 1968 they moved to Miami, and six months later she was dead—"female trouble," he says, back when you couldn't detect it.

He met a widow, Min, who lived a few doors away. They began taking nightly walks on the beach, holding hands. She made him his favorite breakfast, lox and eggs, and told him any movie he wanted to see was fine by her. She was a dancer, with the same legs now that she had as a kid; she kept that figure until the day she died. She intuited his thoughts almost before he had them, acted before his body gathered the nerve. One night they were in her house watching TV. He leaned in to kiss her, looped his arm around the curve of her shoulder. Abruptly she stood, and he lost his grasp. She pulled him up, facing him, walking backward to her room, and at the click of the door she revealed herself, piece by piece, the soft rasp of her skirt hitting her blouse hitting her bra the only sounds in the room. Every part of his mind shut down, from the sophisticated to the puerile, and he could not generate one thought that his body might hear and obey. It remained wholly still, trapped inside itself, unable even to tremble. She looked at him; he looked down at himself. The room bulged with his failure. "Don't worry, Herman," she said. "We have time."

Is it crazy—even dangerous—to feel like a kid again, to be as thrilled and terrified as he was his very first time? Here is Margot, sweet, sassy Margot, finally giving in to his granite kisses and lurching embrace, moving, ever so slowly, cautiously, from the matching club chairs to her bed, the sleek ceramic cats perched atop her armoire keeping curious watch, and all he can think about is what happened nearly eighty years ago, back in 1930, when he was seventeen and foolish and decided, one summer night, to take a train from the Bronx to somewhere in New Jersey. There were five of them, Herman and four of his best friends, and they walked close in a pack, taking and giving one another's heat, reciting aloud the street names, counting down the house numbers. There it was, and the door opened, unleashing delicate fronds of smoke and the metallic scent of sweat. A girl beckoned—she couldn't have been much older than he—and he followed the pendulum taunt of her rear as she climbed the stairs. A click of the door, the rasp of piling material, and a voice scything through the quiet: "One dollar," she said, and his fingers shook when they scraped her palm. "I got on top of her," he remembers, "and I was so excited, instead of going in her, I came outside of her, all over her." The girl hoisted herself to her elbows. "Give me another dollar," she said, "and I'll give you the best you ever had." Couldn't she tell, he thought, that he'd never had *any*? He surrendered another dollar, and it happened all over again. Sorry, no refund. Next time, he stayed in Manhattan, visiting a whorehouse on West Seventy-ninth Street, and got a blow job instead.

So now here's a truth it will always take a lifetime to discover: your last time is no easier than your first. Margot is yielding to him, casting off her blazer, stepping out of her slacks, kicking her orthopedic stilettos across the floor. He does what she likes best, and caresses her arm, gently, with studied focus, as if that were the only part of herself she cared to offer. His dentures graze her neck. He finds her lips, whisks his tongue inside her mouth. They tousle in slow motion; her artfully arranged hair doesn't move. His hands know well what they're doing, "touching her breasts, touching her behind, maybe even going a little further than that." His fingers move with experience, now, with precision, and he feels that she's "enjoying it, enjoying it very much"—a passionate girl, his Margot, in all senses of the word, for better or for worse. It is hard to get hard now, there's no other way to say it, but his body knows the stakes and anticipates the reward: a few minutes, maybe, a timid climax with scant evidence, the pale but prideful hope that he will earn his place in her memories. Something melancholy in the capture, at once a brilliant awakening and irrevocable loss. She lets him find her and there is nothing between them now, not the slim, uncertain wedge of their futures, nor the long tangled sprawl of their pasts.

Somewhere I Have Never Traveled, Gladly

Meghan O'Rourke

When I was sixteen, my mother sat me down at the dining room table and told me, "You can never do anything this year as bad as what I did when I was sixteen." She said it as a warning, leaning forward in her chair. I had been cutting classes, smoking cigarettes (she found a pack in my coat pocket), and developing a "bad attitude."

I took the warning as a challenge. How could I not?

I was a junior in high school, and I was unhappy because I had been dumped the previous summer by an older student—"seventeen going on thirty," as my father would moodily describe him—with whom I had decided not to have sex. (I was a young fifteen.) A month later, he had sex with another girl. A month after that, he broke up with me, shruggingly saying he was not that into girls at the moment. Now I was recklessly trying to achieve some level of sophistication, a quality I had been indifferent to a year ago. Beset by existential dread, I took acid one day, wearing my mother's old halter-top summer dress. With my best friend, I read Sylvia Plath and drank bitters and lemonade; on a lonely afternoon, I went to an East Village gallery to look at bleached-out photographs of

Jesus figures crucified in suburban backyards. Once, coming home high from Roosevelt Island in the middle of the night, I got lost on a subway and wandered through the fluorescent cars, consulting my watch as if it would help. Would I ever get home again?

For a while, scared by my emptiness, I dated a straight-arrow friend who couldn't understand why I was skipping calculus for the second time that week. I didn't want to be a good girl anymore. I wanted to smoke and drink and have migraines and talk late into the night about Baudelaire and the Replacements, and, above all, I wanted not to be a child.

I thought my mother's words that day were a challenge I could meet. Sixteen years later, I think she was right. I couldn't do anything like she did when she was sixteen. While she was still a student, my mother ran off with a teacher at her Catholic high school. That teacher is my father. My mother met him when she was sixteen (I think) and he was twenty-two.

A straight-A student, the oldest of six in a traditional Irish Catholic family, she was caught in class one day writing a letter to her then-boyfriend about smoking pot with some friends. It was the late 1960s; she was a junior. The changes that were stirring up the country had reached suburban New Jersey towns like the one where my mother grew up. Even good Catholic girls like my mother, who dressed in brown saddle shoes and proudly displayed her merit badge on her sweater, were swept up in the shift. Whip-smart, bored, she wasn't quite tuning in and turning on, as the phrase went, but she was lighting up in more ways than one. I imagine, though she never said this, that she observed that many young women around her became housewives and spent the days doing errands and defrosting meat, while the men around her got to have careers and influence. I imagine she found the first prospect unsettling.

Enter my father.

After the nuns confiscated the letter, my mother was distraught:

Her strict, conventional father would not be happy when he learned what it said. One of her friends said, "You should talk to that young new Latin teacher, Mr. O'Rourke; he might be able to help you." My father was just out of college and had returned home to teach for a year or two before finding his way out of the suburbs. My mother was beautiful, with dark hair and an aquiline nose. (In pictures from the time, she looks like Ali McGraw, except perhaps prettier.) I imagine he took a look at her and decided to help. Was the letter in an envelope? he asked. Was it addressed? Yes. Then the nuns had no right to open it; that was mail fraud. And with this, his rebellious sense of justice was awakened.

The nuns agreed not to call my grandfather.

That summer, my mother and father began meeting up, ostensibly to study Greek together.

In my father, my mother immediately saw someone who could challenge her. She once told me that she married my father because he was the smartest man she'd ever met. He was a college graduate, a Latin scholar, a bit of a rebellious wiseass. Though they grew up in towns separated only by a river, Middletown and Red Bank, and both came from Irish Catholic families with six children, the similarities largely stopped there. My father's home was self-consciously intellectual: filled with books, wine, the sound of opera; the walls were covered with prints of ancient Italy, whereas my mother grew up in a family characterized more by warmth and witty chatter; its hearth, appealingly, was the pool out back where my mother's many sisters and their friends congregated.

The tutorial quickly devolved to my parents driving around in my dad's car, smoking pot, or parking on a dirt road near a horse farm to sit under a tree for hours.

One thing led to another.

Like most scandalous family stories, my parents' story did not arrive intact. My brother and I had to sniff it out in pieces. Growing up, I always yearned for my parents to have a romantic story like the ones I read in books. One day, when I was ten, my friend Marian called me up, an air of intrigue in her voice.

I could tell she was dying to tell me something.

"Did you know your parents eloped?" she finally asked.

At this point, *elope* was to me a thrilling word. It sounded like something a mysterious gazelle or eland might do—at once ethereal and passionate. I made a disbelieving sound.

"Eloped!" she continued. "Your father was a teacher at your mother's school and they ran away together! They had an affair and were discovered and *ran away*. Stanley told my mother." (Stanley was a friend of my parents.) I was confused, but I believed her: Marian had always been the one who knew adult secrets. (In the second grade, in the classroom loft, she asked me, "Do you know where babies come from?" I paused, sensing a complicated answer. "SEX!" she whispered.)

The story trickled down to us bit by bit, usually when my parents had had an extra glass of wine. First my mother told me she was married at nineteen; then eighteen; then, finally, seventeen. At Easter one year, my mother and her sisters made margaritas, and as the lunch grew festive, Joanne, the second oldest, said, "But nothing beats when Barbara snuck off every day at Cape Cod to see Paul . . ." and we heard the story of how my mother got my father to come to Cape Cod the same week that her family was going, and then invented a friend, Mary Jane, whom she'd met on the beach, and whom she would go to "play with" every day. This plan backfired: my parents found out. My aunts laughed uproariously as they told the story. It is a funny story, a good story—a story about family and surviving and surprise. But it was also odd to be sixteen listening to stories of your mother's sexual exploits—with a teacher. The parental pretense that sexuality doesn't exist, that it is something I should be careful about, had gone up in a whiff of smoke, drained like the dregs of a margarita, as my mother told her sisters to stop, covered my ears, laughing, clearly enjoying herself.

She was a bad girl, I see. And I also see that she still likes the memory.

But I don't get the whole story until soon after I turned seventeen, when I have my first serious boyfriend, M. I've just graduated from high school, and my parents and M. and I are out celebrating at an Italian restaurant. In love as the young tend to be, fiercely, narcissistically, M. and I have been, for three months, all over each other—"Nice neck arrangement," my English teacher says to me one day, and I don't know if she means my plastic green beaded necklace or the blooming red mark on my neck. I just remember the nervy, jangling feeling of being in love and seeing the world through parallel eyes for the first time. I remember walking along the street near his parents' house, smelling honeysuckle in the air, thinking I would never be elated in this way again. His parents had read an e. e. cummings poem at their wedding, and one day he read me cummings (like so many adolescents in love). It seemed to capture the novel (to us) erotic atmosphere through which we moved:

> somewhere i have never travelled, gladly beyond
> any experience, your eyes have their silence:
> in your most frail gesture are things which enclose me,
> or which i cannot touch because they are too near
>
> your slightest look easily will unclose me
> though i have closed myself as fingers,
> you open always petal by petal myself as Spring opens
> (touching skilfully, mysteriously) her first rose

That summer night, at an Italian restaurant with my parents', there's a charge in the air, a nostalgic alertness. We are nearly the same age they were; we have the same grave sense that our love is not a mere adolescent romance, that it has a depth that will be hard to replicate as the years go on. M. and I recently had sex for the first time, in my parents' bed—ostensibly, because I had a twin mattress—one weekend when they were away. Looking back, I am struck by the Freudian oddness of it all, struck by how innocently (is that the word?) children model themselves on their own parents, even when it comes to sex, with all its incestuous implications. That night, they tell us about how they met, sneaking off into a world of their own making, convinced no one else's rules were right for them. It resonates with us. M.'s therapist is sure our relationship is going to end soon, when we are separated by college, but I, at least, am still persuaded it will last forever. And so we take comfort—encouragement—from my parents, as if we *are* them, or will be.

But we weren't them. I loved M., but part of me felt I was losing myself. My interest in him sometimes seemed like a negation; in darker moods, it seemed to pose a threat to my autonomy, my need to be a person who could make her own choices. We broke up at the end of my freshman year in college.

My parents' story is romantic. But it is also a story of sex, of impermissible sexual attraction, for all that it may also have had an intellectual component; in my father's brilliance, in his education and interests, my mother saw a world beyond frozen vegetables and dinette tables and the limits of her Catholic school. Whatever we call this connection, it pushed against all social forces that wished it to go away and insisted on creating a world, the world we, their children, grew up into, a world that was ours and yet remained somehow exclusively theirs. Like lovers in the garden naming the world, they renamed each other. She became "Kelly" or "Kel" rather than "Barbara." He was "Pablo" rather than "Paul." Channeling his inner Irish aristocracy, he began signing his letters to her "the Prince of Breiffni," which was, in fact, his rightful title, if you followed his family's genealogy back to before Oliver Cromwell burnt the family's castle down to its foundations—four hundred years ago.

It is peculiar to grow up and into a story like this one. What seems like your staid family becomes your strange family. You exist because of a risk taken, heeded, hewed to. The risk, of course, is sexual. After all, the relationship my parents had would not now be condoned by any institution or family. While most things that gave Catholic parents pause in 1966 (birth control, sexual content in movies or books, etc.) are now part of popular culture, this one is not. The idea of a twenty-something college graduate having sex with a sixteen-year-old girl would seem worse now than it did then; then, at least, more women got married young, and political correctness and the work of second-wave feminists hadn't made us hyperaware of the fraught power dynamics in such a relationship—hadn't made us more concerned with safety than with freedom.

Even so, their affair carried its risks for my mother. She would tell me how she nearly didn't graduate from Barnard, so caught up was she in her married life. I remember seeing how inflected her coming-of-age was by my father's sense of himself; she told me about being intimidated by his friends when she first moved to New York. For some reason, it made me nervous about ever being beholden to a man.

All loves come to an end, even when we don't want them to. Last Christmas, my mother died after two years of "battling" cancer and almost forty years of being married to my father. In her last months, my father had found it difficult to go to the hospital with her for doctor's appointments. I didn't understand it. Then two nights before she died, while she was home in hospice care, I woke up on the couch to see that my father had come down the stairs and was standing in his sweatshirt, looking at her in the darkness, fists punched into his sweatshirt pouch, shoulders hunched; he stood like this for minutes, gazing down on her sleeping face.

She died on Christmas Day. Two nights later, I saw M. again. There is a truism, dating back to something Freud observed in "Mourning and Melancholia," that grief makes you either sexually voracious or frigid. I'm not sure either applied to me, but I can say that in the month around my mother's death a strange thing happened: I became preoccupied with M. We had run into each other in a coffee shop a year earlier. Shortly before my mother died, we began to go out now and then, and one night we kissed over dinner. It was eerie, like standing with one foot in the past and one in the present. He smelled the same. The pleasure of being with him again contained an undertow of sadness: to look at him was to feel all the time that had passed, and also how our deepest impressions of the world run just below the surface of our mind like a humming electric wire, there to be touched at any time, capable of shocking us into feeling. Half out of my mind as I was with grief, it spoke to me.

Two days after my mother died, M. came up to Connecticut, where my parents lived. He arrived on an afternoon train, laden with bagels. I had not eaten a meal since my mother died, and after he toasted them we ate them thick with cream cheese and lox, and then, like teenagers, went to the basement rec room and hung out with my college-age brother, watching TV. It was comforting, this re-creating of childhood innocence, this hiding from the upstairs, as if we could go back through time. I felt like I was made of glass. I sat next to M. carefully, leaving a gap between us. That's right, he murmured. God forbid you touch me. And in that moment my younger self flooded back. I laughed; the first moment of solace since my mother had died.

That night, we slept together in a dark room that seemed darker than any I had known. In *The New Black,* the British psychoanalyst Darian Leader notes that "promiscuity and dissipation are simply mechanisms of denial. We search frantically for substitutes for the lost loved one, to obliterate our feelings of loss." It's funny to read these clinical words months later, seeing how they describe dispassionately a chaos that is so threatening, so overwhelming, it seems only another's body can help assuage it. In this case, it was as if, somehow, in being with him, I were my mother, being a seventeen-year-old again, as if I had made *her* decision, and that could bring her back. I was also aware that we were enacting a scene I had seen many times over—maybe once, even, in a movie I had watched with him, when we were seventeen: there is a funeral, and a woman and a man in a car, and they have sex in the car on the way back from the graveyard to the family. How odd. Now, improbably, after all that time apart, we were those people; that emotion the film captured, the black hole inside, was now in *me*.

We saw each other a few more times after that. Perhaps fittingly, the last time I saw him was at my mother's memorial service.

We all know, in some abstract way, how our parents' sexuality inflects ours; but we often talk about it obliquely, laughingly invoking Freud and taboos, or keeping such thoughts for a therapist's office. My parents' story was a romance in the classical sense, but it was also, from another perspective, a romance novel, steamy, lewd in intervals. If it had had a different ending, it would have seemed more troubling, but because it had the right kind of ending—they lived happily ever after, sort of—it became a romance. As it got told, collectively, in its fragments over the years, the story is bittersweet. They are found out and forbidden to see each other. My father loses his job at the Catholic school; my mother is sent to the public school. She applies to college as a junior and is accepted to Barnard. She elopes with my father—yes, elopes—joining him in New York in an apartment against the wishes of her parents. My mother is sixteen or seventeen, I am not sure. They are always evasive on this point. Never mind that the marriage might be said to have erased the crime. One day—"it was a beautiful day, the most beautiful day you could imagine," my mother told me two months before she died—my mother's father was driving to work when he had a heart attack. A few minutes later, he was dead.

My mother told her mother she didn't have to get married. Her mother said: No. You are going to get married—here in our backyard. The wedding pictures are square black-and-white photos with crimped edges. My father is—for once—in a suit, his hair at an awkward length, curling strangely around his ears. My mother is beautiful in a white lace dress and Spanish veil.

It seems to me that all these intersections, of romance, of love, get at something larger than just my family's story. They get at a kernel of a truth about how quickly the role of love and sex shifted in young women's lives. At seventeen, I was frightened of love because I found it potentially limiting. At seventeen, my mother was excited by love, because she found it expansive, eye-opening. It brought her out of suburban New Jersey and into Brooklyn and Barnard in the 1970s, at a time when young writers and artists were first congregating in the borough. She had children and became an educator. I feared that love would hold me back. Like many liberal-minded women of my generation, I thought it was my birthright to be sexually free in my twenties. The frames we came to sex and romance with led us to make radically different choices. Who knows if either was better; the point is just that we make choices, and then we live them out. That is life. Volition is really only a small part of the whole.

It was harrowing to see M. in those weeks near my mother's death. Perhaps that's why I wanted to. To remember what it was to be sixteen trying to become adult, to see sex as the gateway to an adulthood just out of reach—and to remember the grace of falling in love, of finding a person who took me "somewhere I have never travelled, gladly," much as with my father my mother went somewhere she had never traveled, gladly—to Brooklyn, to a world of Szechuan food, drafty brownstones, painters and writers and teachers, conversation and children.

It is of course discomfiting to write this account. These words still feel too frontal to me, too unironic, too cerebral to capture the dark spaces and silences, the night hours that shape our ideas of need. Putting into words any theory about my mother and myself is to turn the complexity of our experiences into a single narrative, rather than the loom of fine threads it is. As I finish, it occurs to me that perhaps that's why Cummings writes "somewhere I *never* travelled." Desire, love, these are places we cannot map and fail to return from, so that they live within us below the surface: our Neverlands.

Skin, Just Skin

A Dramatic Triologue

Eve Ensler

(To be performed by Three Women)

WOMAN 1:   Sometimes it's so can't stop
Take off shirt
Undo belt
Clumsy
You do it
No, I'll do it
Undo bra
One more hook
Strip down

WOMAN 2:   Sometimes it's all about
Skin just skin
Just the way skin

WOMAN 3:   Oh God, sometimes it's like mouth on mouth
Teeth
Tongue
Have to

WOMAN 1:   Sometimes

It's accidental
You thought you were friends
And this current
Turns into one week
In a small hotel room in East Berlin.

WOMAN 2: Oh, nice. Who was that?

WOMAN 3: Sometimes it's
About watching

WOMAN 2: Or being watched
Undressing in front of him
In front of the big window

WOMAN 1: Sometimes it's you putting a hand
On yourself
And him watching
And Rome watching him
Watching

WOMAN 2: Sometimes
It's a crowded boat filled
With cheering tourists
On the Adriatic
As you're both caught there
Naked humping in the sand
And you don't stop

WOMAN 1: You didn't stop?

WOMAN 3: Sometimes it's scuff marks on the off-yellow carpet
In the posh South Kensington apartment

WOMAN 2: Sometimes it's a dare
Forty-five floors up
Mouth on him
In a building that once existed
And he comes by the time

WOMAN 1: Oh God, I always dreamed of doing that

WOMAN 3: Sometimes it's driving on the mad
Italian speedway at a thousand miles
Your face buried in his jeans

WOMAN 1: Sometimes it's a melting hot
Summer day and you're passed out
In the afternoon
And you wake up with his rugged face
Between your legs

WOMAN 2: Sometimes it's a work night
And you get home early
And you take a bath
And undress
And play with yourself
Lying there casual and stark naked
On the bed
And you're on your knees before she remembers
It's been a hard day

WOMAN 3: I didn't know you were with women . . . when was
that?

WOMAN 1: Sometimes it's the twenty-nine-year-old thin boy
From the village
With the curly black hair
Who comes to your summer house
On the edge of the sea
And kisses you and you know it's August
And you're suddenly not fifty-four

WOMAN 3: Sometimes it's a song

WOMAN 2: Or a joint

WOMEN 123: Or too much chocolate

WOMAN 1: Sometimes it's only chocolate

WOMAN 2: Or birthday cake at midnight
Because one of you is married

WOMAN 3:   No, you didn't

WOMAN 2:   I didn't. I wanted to, but I didn't

WOMAN 3:   Sometimes he just says do you mind
            If I kiss you and it occurs to you that you don't
            And you end up with your mouth on his for
            eight hours and
            The sun comes up

WOMAN 1:   Sometimes you wake up and he's inside
            You and your body is more aroused 'cause it's
            So early and you're so
            Sleepy and nothing has ever felt like that

WOMAN 3:   Sometimes it's that window
            Wide open in Montauk
            And it's so bright you're
            Only wearing sunglasses
            Looking out
            As he takes you from behind
            Sweating and screaming out

WOMAN 2:   And sometimes
            It just happens in Portugal
            For the first time in seven years
            You find each other
            And you're not afraid

WOMAN 1:   Sometimes it's the hysteria that comes
            After he has been that deep inside you
            And the crying is a way of coming

WOMAN 2:   And sometimes
            It's riding him like a bronco

WOMAN 3:   Or humping her like you're about to get there

WOMAN 1:   And sometimes it's the three of you in a hot tub
            And you end up entangled not knowing
            Whose hair whose mouth whose hand

WOMAN 2:	And sometimes you dress up
	And they take it off you
WOMAN 3:	Sometimes it's hardness
WOMAN 2:	It's softness
WOMAN 1:	It's grabbing
WOMAN 2:	It's refusing
WOMAN 3:	It's dangerous
WOMAN 1:	Embarrassing
WOMAN 2:	Sometimes it's
	"You're beautiful"
WOMAN 3:	or
	"God, your ass"
WOMAN 2:	"Your skin"
WOMAN 1:	And sometimes it's so insanely funny
	It's ridiculous

(They all become hysterical)

WOMAN 2:	But mainly it takes longer
	It's all preparation
WOMAN 3:	You lose track of who begins
WOMAN 1:	Who's on top
WOMAN 2:	Who got more
WOMAN 3:	Who's inside who

Reading of *O*

Honor Moore

1.

I avoided it. Never even saw a copy of it all those years. But it lay there, beneath my young woman feminism. A curiosity. A taboo.

Written by a woman, I heard. To entertain her husband.

A friend of mine met her in Paris. Pauline Réage. She was small, a literary woman who wore glasses. She came into the room, her face obscured by a hat.

The marvelous name was a nom de plume.

2.

In a dark apartment near St. Germain, a woman hands a sheaf of pages to a man wearing a suit.

3.

I had returned to the city after years in the country and for a few months lived in a loft at the border of Little Italy and SoHo. I was writing and it was winter, and as snow fell outside I described it. Meticulously. How it fell on the roof of the church across the street. How it dulled a red door that led from the roof to god knows where.

How something that had looked yellow in sunlight in falling snow had no color whatsoever.

I was having a love affair after years of involuntary abstinence. I was still "a woman" I had discovered.

I thought of myself as in the process of having a sexual awakening. I thought of myself as "a girl at fifty."

4.

The first time I was alone with him, we stood at a small distance from each other and I trembled. When I saw him again I scarcely recognized him. It was not how he looked that had caused me to tremble.

Because circumstances proscribed the dimensions of the affair, restraint became its method. For instance, he never came to see me in that loft at the borders of SoHo and Little Italy.

Or lie with me in that bed. It was built of dark wood and highly polished, the bedclothes were white, and its surface stood high, at an unusual height from the floor.

5.

One night after seeing the film based on Proust's *Time Regained,* I returned alone to the loft. I had in mind to choose a book, and there it was. *Story of O.* I pulled it from the shelf: on the white cover, a characterization by Eliot Fremont-Smith of the *New York Times*: "A total, authentic literary experience."

The critic's name brought back the room where I began to write in 1972. The American edition had appeared in 1965, the year I lost my virginity.

In the country I had lived alone and taken care of an old house. Which made me strong, as did writing a long book. By the time I moved back to the city, I was weary of my strength and its requirements.

6.

" . . . they notice, at one corner of the park, at an intersection where there are never any taxis, a car which, because of its meter, resembles a taxi.

Get in, he says.

She gets in. . . ."

7.

Even now, without the book in hand, I can see the cool interior of that automobile, the green of trees through the window as the driver makes his way out of the city. Also, I have the sensation of the leather upholstery, how it sticks to the nakedness of her buttocks.

And can recall the feel of the man sitting next to her.

8.

Now a man wearing a mask is entering the woman's cell in the château at Roissy. With chains, he secures her wrists to the wall above her bed. And fits her neck with a wide leather collar.

The mechanisms are mercilessly described. "They had clasps, which functioned automatically like a padlock when it closes, and they could be opened only by means of a small key."

The click of her mules as she walks the tiled corridors, her pale flesh reflecting the fire in the hearth of the library where she is presented, the men with their drinks circling her, making their crude remarks. And then she is whipped.

9.

I feel myself abruptly frantic, a woman enraged at being kept from her pleasure. I toss the book aside.

Hot blur of white bedclothes, black night out the window, the burning, my own fists pounding the mattress beside me, the rising torso, a fury of moaning no one can hear, so thick are the walls of the old loft building, and afterward the fumbling for it, the book written by a woman in Paris when I was a child, its yellowed pages beneath the reading lamp.

Again and again.

10.

Which shocked me.

11.

She wears the taffeta gown caught up at the waist: in the back to reveal her buttocks, in the front to expose her "belly."

She is not the only woman in the château, and she is not permitted to speak to the others, nor they to her. Like the others, she is directed to keep her eyes lowered, and if she meets the gaze of any of the men who "use" her, she is beaten.

The word "mule" and the idea of that kind of unsecured shoe enter my erotic imagination.

Riding crop. The whip with several knotted lashes. The one fashioned of bamboo and leather.

It is the year 2000, and there is no talk of torture in the news.

12.

If I were a feminist critic, I would note the narrator's presence at the opening of the novel, as in: "Then, when her blindfold was removed, she found herself standing alone in a dark room, where they left her for half an hour or an hour, or two hours, I can't be sure . . ."

I would put forth *Story of O* as a novel with a marriage plot, in which the heroine chooses self-actualization over domesticity.

Or the narrative of a saint's life that culminates in martyrdom.

13.

When I have watched pornographic films, I have been aroused but also disgusted, but no matter how "disgusting" the events that befall O, her story does not disgust me.

As she bent, I bent. As she prepared, I prepared. As she was beaten, I was beaten. As she was fucked, I was fucked. As she was denied, I made her accommodation.

14.

" . . . O tried to figure out why there was so much sweetness mingled with the terror in her, or why her terror seemed itself so sweet. . . ."

15.

Such is the understanding of sexuality—as something beyond good and evil, beyond love, beyond sanity; as a resource for ordeal and for breaking through the limits of consciousness—that informs the French literary canon that I have been discussing.

Story of O, with its project for completely transcending personality, entirely presumes this dark and complex vision of sexuality so far removed from the hopeful view sponsored by American Freudianism and liberal culture. The woman who is given no other name than O progresses simultaneously toward her own extinction as a human being and her fulfillment as a sexual being.

—SUSAN SONTAG, 1967

16.

One Christmas I dined in the restaurant in Paris, where, in a private dining room, Sir Stephen had shared O with two other men.

17.

It must have been dawn when I finished the book, but I do not remember the light or whether it was still snowing.

"Down on your knees," says my lover on the telephone.

Trembling, I picture myself there.

And then we laugh.

Going All the Way

Liz Smith

In 1939, my birthplace in Texas wasn't the metropolis complex that it is today—a huge hub for international travel with museums, art galleries, fashion, insurance, oil, and the cattle "bidness" at the center of it.

Back in the 1930s, Fort Worth was still a small town, complete with streetcars and a uniformed cop on every other corner. The country had begun emerging inch by inch from the Great Depression that had crushed America after the stock market crashed in 1929.

Even insular Texans were beginning to be aware that this was a dangerous world and a bunch of thugs called the Nazis were about to march into Poland and throw the world into chaos. I even recall some months later, my high school class experienced our French teacher, weeping that the Germans had paraded down the Champs-Elysées in Paris. We cried with her, for Paris was a city of our dreams where American talents such as F. Scott Fitzgerald, Ernest Hemingway, and Gertrude Stein abounded and impressionist art reigned supreme. We knew about Paris—it was where women danced bare-breasted in the Follies Bergère.

On the other hand, life in Fort Worth was provincial and insular, full of misplaced western pride and obsessions with football. Racism and southern paternalism still beset the great state of Texas (Lyndon Johnson's civil rights advances lay far in the future) . . . A demagogue Catholic priest, Father Coughlin, was forever on the radio preaching hatred. (There was no such thing as being politically correct.) We didn't listen; we preferred Walter Winchell, Jack Benny, and "The First Nighter" hurrying to his seat in the little radio theater off Times Square. . . . Women had not joined the workforce as they would when World War II became a terrible fact of life. In fact, women were still second-class citizens, having only won the vote nineteen years earlier.

It was a world where my narrow-minded grandmother believed in a hard-shell kind of Baptist religion that frowned upon men and women in bathing suits swimming together and disapproved of ballroom dancing. This was too rigid even for my devout mother. My grandma used to make dresses for her neighbors for two dollars apiece but once turned down a chance where the dress pattern was sleeveless. "No decent woman would wear a sleeveless dress," she opined. (Shades of wardrobe malfunction!) My father was broad-minded, liking jokes, gambling, and dancing. But even he was shocked to see a woman smoking on the streets. And he felt pregnant women should stay at home and not be seen. My mother once said, "*Sex* is the ugliest word in the English language."

We kids thought "sex" was a delicious if forbidden idea. We could read and did read the classics. We had even heard that in France, a woman named Coco Chanel had created a sensation wearing trousers at the beach. Women in pants, in Texas! Never, unless she was contributing to a cattle roundup.

So now you have the idea of my youth in Fort Worth, Texas. Let's now introduce sex and bring us into the present tense.

I'm sixteen. I'm dating for the first time—really. The locale is Fort Worth, Texas, pre-World War II. We drive around in cars, we eat in cars, we neck in cars. We never go "all the way." We girls are more concerned with getting to the famous Fort Worth Casino on Lake Worth, dancing to Tommy Dorsey's visiting orchestra—or somebody else famous on tour. There's a skinny kid fronting for Dorsey; name of Frank Sinatra. He's good and it's all very romantic.

I'm trying to break away from the Southern Baptist environment that has dominated my life. My secret passion for show biz glamour and my family's embedded church life are warring with one another.

On many nights I am double-dating with my favorite cousin, a charming guy who is a little older than I am. I'll call him X in order not to smear the family names. X is cute and funny and snappy, full of jokes and one-liners, a marvelous dancer and storyteller. He always drives the car with one hand and makes the gearshift go into place, manipulating it with his knees. He starts any evening we go out as a foursome by wisecracking, "Well, what do you want to do—first?" I know what he means but I just giggle.

I was always mad about him, but he has really cute adorable girlfriends and he is so appealing. I am invariably more interested in what he's doing in the front seat of the car than I am in whomever I'm with in the backseat. I feel I amount to a big disappointment and I know my dates never measure up, as I'm forever equating them with X.

Comes a soft Texas night when we're not going out. We've had a family picnic in the Smith backyard where our mutual grandparents live. But everyone else—adults and children have segued off to a Wednesday night party at the local church. X and I are just sitting in sling chairs, looking at the starry Texas skies. We're listening to Glenn Miller coming over the radio from the kitchen.

We have ended up side by side, not saying anything. The rest of our cousins, siblings, and adults have gone. "What you say, kiddo?" asks X, lighting a cigarette. (He's too young to smoke but he would live into his eighties anyway, so what did we know back then about the dangers of smoking?)

"I don't know, Bub," I answer. He leans over and kisses me softly on the cheek. This is a far cry from his usually jokey manner. "Ya know, kid, I really love you. We always kid around and we're with other people, but it's you I've got my eye on. They don't know where we are tonight, so let's stay here under the stars and make out."

I am so shocked I can't speak. It's as if he has been reading my tiny mind. "Okay," I say slowly. He gets up, he goes off and comes back with an old quilt and a couple of pillows and spreads them on the ground. He pulls me down on top of him, and I feel him hard against me. I think I might faint. I've been around boys and my brothers all my life, but I've never paid any attention to their fooling around. I guess I didn't want to know too much.

Now I know. X and I start kissing and he really knows how— slow, sweet, and tender. Fabulous. So that's what this is all about? Hmmm, it makes practicing kissing with my girlfriends seem absolutely idiotic.

I keep caressing him back and it's all instinctive. I haven't any idea what the end result will be, but I didn't seem to need a lot of instruction. "Look at me," he whispers. "Look at me. I love you. I want to be inside of you."

And so—it happened. Most virgins report poor results for a "first" time. Not me. I know we didn't use any birth control; didn't think about it. (What fools we sexually uneducated mortals were!) I don't remember if I had an orgasm; I was so ecstatically having "something" special happen that I didn't know if I was missing something else.

When all this passion and friction and mind-blowing was going on, time passed, unnoted. Finally, gasping like fish out of water, we lay back and looked at the stars. Then he said, "That was stupid of me. Next time, we use a rubber."

Next time? Light began to dawn. He was my cousin. My first cousin. There was to be no "next time." And, it never happened again though he tried and tried and I began to do that thing females do. They say no when they mean yes. I just knew that down the road we would create such a mess between our families, it wasn't worth imagining.

Fortunately he soon went off with my older brother to join the air force because the Selective Service Act would happen anyway and they'd be drafted as buck privates. Temptation was removed in the form of patriotism, and the war lasted a long time. But I stayed half in love with him for years and years. He wrote me wonderful letters, and in time, after 1945, he returned to Fort Worth and we became "just cousins" again, seeing each other seldom and off and on in others' company. We met socially at family reunions. Marriages ensued, children, years passed—I grew up. I read Masters and Johnson, *Playboy,* Helen Gurley Brown, and I experienced the Swinging 1960s and every other kind of sexual freedom they had to offer. I developed my personal tastes.

But nothing ever thrilled me like that one night under the stars. He was my "college education." When X was retiring, not too long ago, he wrote me a letter. We had always corresponded without mentioning "it!" "I have never stopped thinking about you and about our night. My marriage is over. I am old now but I am still thinking about you. You need to stop working. Retire and come live with me in Arizona. The best is yet to be!"

He died alone shortly after this. But he has dominated my sexual reveries through all these years. That little experience was so surprising and so wonderful, I'd have to give it an A plus.

I wonder what would have happened if I had retired with him to Arizona.

The Man in Question

Rebecca Walker

The best sex I ever had was sex I never had. I was young, younger than I am now. I was twentysomething, and beautiful. Yes, I say that about myself because it is true. My skin was smooth and unlined. My body was unblemished, fit from Pilates and regular shots of liquid oxygen. I moved with certainty from my strengthened core. My hair, a natural rich brown, shined. I believed in exploration and having fun. My entire life was before me. I was young, much younger than I am now.

I lived in New York. I owned a beautiful apartment. I had a book contract. I had lovers but was in between several at the time. One lived in Russia on a Fulbright. He sent postcards. Another was truly and hopelessly wrong for me. She was poor, or should I say, less well off, and she liked dogs. Big ones. And I did not like dogs. Well, I liked her dogs, but not when they scratched the wood floors of my apartment. I did not like her dogs that much. And anyway, she was wrong for me. But the sex, now the sex, was very, very good. Until that point the best I'd had.

It was sex during which I had to do nothing but recline while she stroked and devoured me, licked and turned me over. She asked for nothing but my satiety. She liked to sneak out just after, leaving me asleep in my bed without herself ever being touched. I woke up the morning after in a daze, stumbling around the apartment, trying to recognize ordinary things like my hairbrush or a pair of running shoes. But she was wrong for me. It is not possible to describe how many ways she was wrong for me. But the sex was so good it is not possible to describe how good it was except to say that I kept having it after realizing she was wrong for me. Except to say we stayed together longer, much longer, than we might have, at least in part because of the sex.

So that is the sex I was having during this period in which I had the best sex I ever had, which was, in fact, sex I didn't have. It was sex I imagined, sex that came frighteningly close to happening. It was sex I wanted but didn't have; I did not let myself be taken.

The man in question lived in an apartment building close to mine and his body was quite appealing—a gentle form, not hard, and yet undeniably masculine. His member, his penis, his dick, was something I imagined I saw even when he wore jeans, and when I did rub myself against it one night, I felt its size and girth and wanted it inside of me. I wanted it inside of me like a girl wants a Popsicle or a piece of dark chocolate, or a fabulous piece of clothing that makes her gasp when she sees herself in the full-length mirror outside of the dressing room. I wanted him and his dick like that and I imagined it countless times.

We were not an item, although he lived one block away and he came over sometimes and we made out hot and heavy in my living room, a room devoid of furniture. And he liked to rub against me, too, and kiss standing up even though I always thought about Robert Doisneau photographs of French lovers at the train station and how cliché they were when we kissed this way. To make it bearable, to make it hot, I pushed him against the wall when we did it that way. I pushed him hard against the wall to feel the flap of his jeans and the tiny copper buttons underneath press against me in the spot I liked, the spot that made me want to fuck him there, in my living room, on the floor with the scratches the dogs made that I was not happy about and which I had called a buffer about because when I thought of fucking this man, I wanted to do it on a smooth floor. I did not want to turn over and see scratches on the floor that would remind me of another person's sex, the way they took me and gave me orgasms that knocked me senseless and left, smug and satisfied by their own proficiency, in the morning.

I want to tell you his name but I can't. He is married with kids now. They live in Santa Barbara, a place I imagine could be sexy, but never as sexy as New York, and in any case, never as sexy as the floor of my apartment in New York on cool autumn nights when the sky turns that exquisite cobalt and all of the city is alive with lights and movement and you are lying beneath a heavy body that you want to devour but you cannot because it is not yours to devour and there is something, something ineffable that keeps you from eating, partaking of the meal.

It was apprehension. Alarms went off in my head when we were together, or when I dialed his number, or met him at a bar. I knew I would like it, his dick, I suppose. That it would be delicious and thus it would ruin me because he was not right for me either, but if I fell in love with his dick, if our fucking became something I could not, or would not, control or do without then I was doomed. That, and also he had been in a relationship with someone I knew. I didn't know her well but still it seemed unethical, wrong somehow, even though I knew she wouldn't mind. She was off to other men, other lands.

The breaking point was this: I was at his house. I was on his bed. These were the days before iPods and he was playing CDs. They were jazz CDs, CDs I liked. He had dimmers on his lights, which I also liked, and which bathed the room in just the exact kind of sophisticated soft, yellow glow that made me feel beautiful. We had come from a small bar deep in the West Village. Did I mention I was young, younger than I am today? I was taut in the right places. The proportion of my curves was just so. His bed was like a woman's bed—perfectly appointed for sex. For luxurious sex. For staying. For never leaving.

He gently coaxed me down onto the bed and it was as lovely as it looked. Down duvet, lovely high-thread-count sheets, soothing colors. It was a cloud of loveliness and then he lay on top of me, reaching up my sweater and pressing against me. He moved slowly, which I liked; he was not a boy you see, he was a man. He was not afraid to go after me, what he wanted, but he wanted also to make me happy, to give me pleasure.

What can I say? I wrapped my legs, still in jeans, a well-fitting pair I had gone to great lengths to find, around his hips and opened my mouth and let his tongue slide against mine. The lights, did I say, were dimmed. Jazz, did I say, perhaps Miles Davis's *Kind of Blue,* played on the CD player. There had been a bit of drinking. Not too much to induce sloppiness, just enough to create a languid sensuality to which we both gave way, because it seemed completely counterintuitive not to, because it felt so good, so fucking right.

I cannot remember why we stopped. A well-intentioned blocking out of an event I didn't want to happen, let alone to relive. I remember only a sudden and abrupt breaking of the closeness, a brutal rent created by something foreign, and intrusive. Was it his brother ringing the bell? Was it my other lover paging me on a tiny beeper, the little black precursor to BlackBerrys and iPhones? Was it again my fear of it being too good, of this man actually being the right fit in bed, in my body, even though he might not be in my life? Was some part of my own life going to be revealed through our fuck? Through the orgasm he did or didn't give me? Through the size of him and the expression on his face when he came? The way he lay with me after? The breakfast we might have? The movie we might then go see, which we may have both liked, at the art house that no longer exists.

Was it too much for me to have something so good: the beautiful boy next door? Perhaps he was not complicated enough because I was beautiful and young and very attached to drama. And there were so many, many things I wanted to do, and this man, I could not be sure where he was going any more than I could be sure where I was going and if I ended up wanting him well then my whole life would change, wouldn't it, and did I really need yet another direction to add to my list? He was the ex-boyfriend of a friend, I was in love with someone else, I was sleeping with another someone else, and I was trying to write a book. All of those things flashed through my mind, which is surprising, because I was young and generally followed my bliss wherever it wanted to take me, no matter how much trouble it caused.

The point, though, is we did stop, and we stopped suddenly. The music went off and the lights went up and I adjusted my top and he said he would walk me home. Yes, yes, I remember it now. His brother came home—they lived together in a postcollege family-dorm kind of way—and there was no privacy. It was a floor-through of a brownstone, and the door between the bedroom and the living room was made of glass. It was, I can see it now, a French door. There was a covering of some sort, but we both decided, silently, each on our own, that to close the curtains would be awkward at best; the brother would know we were inside, on the bed, making love, fucking, having sex, together.

When we reached the door of my apartment building I felt as if every cell in my body pined for release. He could have come upstairs with me. There was my floor, after all, and with or without scratches, it would receive us. I had a Navajo blanket didn't I? I could spread it out and light candles and put on my own music, some women from Mali singing, or from France.

Instead we stayed on the shore. He kissed me in front of the mailboxes. It was a hot and steamy kiss full of promise. All of the signs were there: it would happen. He would penetrate me and I would like it and we would be bound up like that until we were no longer. It was just a matter of time and place and opportunity. We thought this because we were young and did not know the signs. The signs said I was tied up with others and he lived with his brother who came and went and gave him no privacy. The signs said I was afraid to fuck him because I was afraid I would want to fuck him again and again and then what would I do? Would I move in with him? Would we add scratches to my floor with our own love-making? And then perhaps he would leave me, or I would find out he wasn't very bright. I had this notion one night as we talked. Here was someone who knew many things but was not terribly smart. I was a person, I thought at the time, who knew very little but was exceedingly, exquisitely observant. I knew something about the way people moved and what they said with their movements and I knew there was a difference between us, the way we each moved through the world, and I thought to myself yes, this would be an obstacle.

And so we didn't do it. We never did it. But I wanted to do it. I did, I wanted to do it. It was the best sex I ever had, it was the best sex I never had. It is the sex I have replayed over and over in my mind. It is the sex that still sits perched on a ledge, disallowed the jump, the satisfying release, and the rapturous freefall into recovery.

And I think about that man and that bed and that dimmer and that music and that way he pushed my shirt up over my breasts and sucked my nipples until they were harder than they've ever been. I think about the roughness of his clothes brushing up against my bare skin, against the nerve endings there, the ones that made me wet and grab the back of his neck and pull his mouth closer to mine. I think about all of that and I think yes, that is the best sex I've ever had, the sex that lives in my mind, the sex without the messy aftermath, the decisions to be made the next day, the weighing of implications, the ecstasy and then the bitter disappointment. My best sex is the sex that didn't happen, the sex that saved me from opening one door too many.

They Had Sex So I Didn't Have To

Molly Jong-Fast

My mother fought for free love and the right to sexual expression. I fight the traffic as I squire my kids up and down Madison Avenue. Both sets of my grandparents had open marriages. I have a closed marriage (that's where you only sleep with the person you are married to). My mother's mother tells stories of sleeping with my grandfather in the woods and smoking "grass." There are not a lot of woods where I live in Manhattan. If it is every generation's job to swing the pendulum back, then I have done mine.

My father's father (Howard Fast) was famous for his communism, Spartacus, and his various exploits with members of the opposite sex around Hollywood. One of my aunts is known at her prep school for being straight then gay and then straight again. A deceased grandaunt of mine was notorious for being one of the most sexually active octogenarians at The Hebrew Home for the Aged.

And what of my parents? When I was but a young girl I wandered into my eighty-year-old grandfather's bedroom to find on the bedside table the book *Beyond Viagra* staring back at me. Yes, the Jongs, and the Fasts may have little in common but their love of freedom, fear of oppression, and their need for lubrication.

Growing up I knew we were weird. It's hard not to suspect you are weird when you have a Chinese last name but are a redheaded Jew. It's hard not to suspect you are weird when you live in a town house with a hot pink door and a dog called Poochini. And then there was the fact that my mother was always wandering around the house totally nude; this could have been a clue, perhaps.

All this railing against familial nakedness begs the question: am I a prude? Well, I dress like the Orthodox (long skirts, no wig), have been held up by Wendy Shalit as a role model, and have been married (to one man) since I was twenty-four. The short answer would be yes. Yes in the eyes of Erica Jong, I am a prude. (Of course Erica Jong did have a threesome with a certain hideous feminist author who could be described as MC Hammer if MC Hammer were a white lesbian. Portia de Rossi she is not. Hell, Andrea Dworkin she is not.)

The truth is my mother and I grew up in different worlds. My mom was born in 1942, in the middle of World War II. My mother grew up in a world where no one talked about sex. Where sex was secretive and sex was racy. She grew up in a world where sex meant marriage. Where women waited to kiss a boy until they were going steady. My mother grew up in a world where a woman couldn't eat dinner alone in a restaurant, lest she look like a prostitute. She came of age in a universe without easily available birth control, without abortion, without options. My mother wore poodle skirts and twins sets, and had a black-and-white TV. She never witnessed a young Britney Spears pulsating in a bikini musing on her virginity (or lack of).

My nymphomaniacal grandparents were perhaps not typical of their generation, and we cannot discount the effect that my nymphomaniacal grandparents must have had on her.

I grew up in a world that was just the opposite. I grew up in a culture obsessed with sex. My childhood was punctuated by salacious

New York Post headlines. As a girl I remember watching the Anita Hill–Clarence Thomas hearings on CNN. I was sitting in my mom's bedroom, playing with stickers and asking her what a "pube" was.

The 1980s in New York City were a time of contradictions—a time of limousines riding by homeless people, a time of the richest and the poorest as neighbors, living side by side, stealing from the other. The city was boiling with rage, with fear, with crime, and with sex. Sex was everywhere—from sex crimes like the Central Park Jogger case to Donald Trump's divorce from Ivana, to sex clubs like the Vault. Back then pornography was on basic cable (it was on channel J). Sex was everywhere.

Sex was piped into our lives through the media. The library was popular because it housed *Tiger Eyes,* which was the dirtiest of the Judy Blume oeuvre. From books to TV, my teenagehood was hugely influenced by the musings of Aaron Spelling with his *Beverly Hills 90210* and *Melrose Place.* I watched reruns of *Three's Company*— which was filled with innuendo and sexual hijinks that would have been considered pornographic when my mother was a girl. No matter how unsexy a show was, it seemed they always dedicated at least one or two episodes to teen pregnancy or STDs or date rape or some other "sex"-related theme. There was the usual media schizophrenia about sex, but whether it was promoted or profane the topic was still very much in the forefront.

But by 1988 AIDS was just starting to be picked up by the mainstream media. The thing that affected every single girl on the Upper East Side of Manhattan was the AIDS infection of Ally Gertz. Ally Gertz had been a popular girl who had gone to a private school and did everything right . . . Everything right, until she met a cute bartender at Studio 54. She had one one-night stand, and from that she became infected with AIDS. She became a one-woman mission for AIDS awareness. She was a hero, but she was also a victim.

Soon after, someone decided that talking about sex would keep kids from having it, or if they did have it, they would have it safely. People were always asking me if I wanted to talk about sex. I endured hours of school sex education lectures. I went to a very progressive middle school where they had our eighth grade classes go out to the local CVS to buy condoms. The hippy ideal behind this misadventure was that if we were not embarrassed we would be more apt to go off and buy condoms and use them.

My two dorky best friends and I bravely walked down West Eighty-eighth Street. We bravely went into the drugstore. My friend Stephanie was not the type to suffer fools gladly. So as we giggled insanely she took the bull by the horns and bought the prophylactics.

Later we unzipped our backpacks and placed the condoms in the center of the large wooden table. The teacher congratulated us for our courage and ability to remove money from our wallets. We then proceeded to open the condoms and put them on bananas. Even at the tender age of twelve we understood how profoundly misguided our teachers were. We weren't stupid idiots. We knew how to go into a store and buy things. Most of us smoked at least a few cigarettes a day by twelve years old. We weren't short bus riders. Kids have unsafe sex because they think they are invincible not because they are too stupid to buy condoms. It did not create a class of safe-sex zealots, as I think our teachers might have hoped. It did however make sex seem somehow unsexy.

I am my mother's worst bourgeois nightmare. I live on the Upper East Side. I have three children—all by the same man! I never slept with a man who wore cowboy boots. I have never been to a sex club. I have never had a Dominican divorce. I did, however, go to rehab, but that is for "the most drugs I ever had" anthology or possibly "the where did my teens go" anthology. I am a low-rent yuppie, shuttling my children back and forth to the various and sundry activities and involving myself in the Parents' Association. I am the person my grandmother and mother would have watched in silent scorn. I sometimes tell my children that my most important job is taking care of them. I am not saying that I am a better mother than my mother. In fact, I am probably a worse mother than my mother, but I am a more traditional, or should we say, repressed mother than my mother. For example, in this book the great and talented Julie Klam tells her daughter to call her vagina her front. She shows this as an example of her repression. I call this an example of her brilliance.

Maybe I would have been more slutty, if I hadn't grown up watching my mother saunter around our town house au natural, past the pictures of naked lesbians fooling around. Or maybe it was all the book readings I went to growing up. Or possibly it was the trauma of sitting through my mother's fourth wedding and listening to my mother call my stepfather a "horny Boy Scout." It was a phrase I did not soon forget. In fact it still haunts me to this day.

There is also a slim but real chance that this is just who I am. That growing up surrounded by sex did not make me a prude. Though it is true that my mother's generation needed to rebel, to free themselves. Whereas my generation was already free. There was no need for us to fight the power because we were the power. We were the advertising dollars that the consumer goods industry fought for. We had all the rights we needed and possibly more. We didn't need to fight for birth control. We didn't need to fight for the right to choose. We didn't need to fight for the right to vote. There was no reason for us to feel guilty about having sex before marriage. There was nothing to fight against. We didn't need to burn our bras, so we burnt our CDs. And perhaps that's why I'm neither a lover nor a fighter.

Kiss

A Short, Short Story

Erica Jong

We had known each other for twenty years. There had always been electricity between us. But we were friends not lovers. We loved to flirt, to come to the brink and part. He lived in Rome and I in New York.

We first met because we had the same gallery. It was owned by a woman with sour crimson lips who always seemed to be sucking a lemon. Her mother had named her Hermione. She hated it and changed it to Hermes—the name of her gallery. She was tall, had a big nose, and wore outlandish hats—priceless creations of felt and feathers that looked like flying raptors. Her nails were long and bloody. Her perfume was an overpowering mixture of tuberose and jasmine, privately blended.

But she knew how to bring the best critics in—if there is such a thing in critics. And though she took an obscene percentage (50 percent plus expenses) she got the highest prices.

When I met Lorenzo he was married and he still is married—but to a different wife. When I met him I was married to X and now I am married to Y. But none of that matters to the story.

I didn't like his work though it sold ferociously. He made enormous sculptures of roly-poly beasts—bulbous Bambis, obese dancing bears, inflated blue Babars.

At that time I was doing canvases of cunts—open cunts, closed cunts, bleeding mutilated cunts. It was the 70s. I was a guerrilla—and also gorilla—girl.

He pretended to love my work and I pretended to love his. Actually, he loved my breasts and I longed for his huge unseen penis.

How did the kiss begin?

We were in Palm Beach with our spouses. There was a large party made by some billionaire on his five-hundred-foot yacht. Lorenzo and I were wandering about, looking at the Picassos, Braques, the Koonses, the Boteros, when suddenly in the dark of the titanic teak deck he kissed me. That kiss was a promise. It lingered fizzily like a jazz riff. It tongued my clit without touching it. It gave me chills and hots simultaneously. It changed us. From then on we knew there was something more between us.

But his new wife was fiercely jealous; they seldom spent nights apart. She had been married to a player—her second marriage to the corrupt Italian politician—and she was wary. She told Lorenzo if he ever cheated they were through.

Lorenzo was not a beautiful man. He had wild, kinky orange hair and a reddish salt-and-pepper beard. He had huge agate eyes and an aquiline nose and he was not tall but he exuded sex. You knew this man loved sex and appreciated women. You just knew. If I could bottle that, I'd be rich.

The kiss changed the equation. When he next came to New York he set himself up in a downtown penthouse hotel suite with a sauna and a built-in lap pool. He invited me over.

In the elevator, panic struck. I knew that if we consummated this flirtation something would shiver between us, possibly even tip over our marriages, but I pretended not to be scared.

He greeted me with vintage champagne and fresh chocolate-covered cherries. We ate and drank and spoke haltingly. Then we retreated to the couch, wrapped our arms around each other, and began to kiss. It was a kiss that went back to the birth of the universe, the making of the stars, the sculpting of humans out of clay. It was a mitochondrial kiss in which generations were born, died, and were buried, in which trees leaped out, bloomed, fell and rotted, and gave birth to new forests. It was a kiss that moistened oceans, grew the universe, swirled through the cosmos. His tongue, my lips, my tongue, his lips, everything merged in the waters of the womb of his mother, the penis of his father, the souls of his grandparents.

A kiss can be an IOU, or the end of a love affair. A kiss can last for eons. A kiss can be longer and stronger than a fuck. A kiss has a history and a future.

But what was its future? In the first ending we go to bed, are deeply disappointed, and never see each other again.

In the second ending, we go to bed, discover lifelong passion, and turn our lives upside down, saddening spouses, children, parents. But I have chosen an alternate ending. I get up from the couch, run to one of the many glamorous marble bathrooms to pee, dress quickly, then I sneak out the door of the suite.

Now I can keep his kiss for the rest of my life.

Acknowledgments

Thanks to the indefatigable Amanda Lensing, my assistant for word processing, research, appointments, et cetera; Julia Cheiffetz, living proof that Barnard girls are the brainiest and cutest; Katie Salisbury, who works her butt off; Barbara Victor, who read proofs with me and lived through the crises; Bob Miller, who persuaded me with great enthusiasm; Amy Berkower, who thought *Why not?* and did the contract with you know who.

Kisses to my live-in lawyer, KDB. Every writer should sleep with a lawyer—especially in the age of Amazon, if not amazons.

And to my contributors: Hugs, kisses, and no more fear. Women who write about sex *still* get no respect—but we don't give a damn!

—EMJ, March 2011, New York City, my hometown.

(I'd rather be in Rome.)

Contributors

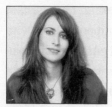

Karen Abbott was born and raised in Philadelphia, where she attended sixteen years of Catholic school—a tenure that gave her an appreciation for all things Magdalene and a finely tuned sense of guilt. Her first book, the *New York Times* bestseller *Sin in the Second City,* tells the true story of two sisters who ran the world's most famous brothel. *American Rose,* her portrait of the legendary Gypsy Rose Lee, was published in January 2011 in honor of the ecdysiast's 100th birthday. She often gives her job description as "Chronicler of Whores and Strippers" and feels as if she were born several generations too late.

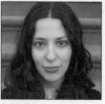

Elisa Albert is the author of *The Book of Dahlia,* a novel, and *How This Night Is Different,* a collection of short stories. She believes reading good sex writing is liberating and that women have a lot of catching up to do in owning our sexuality and doesn't think she needs to apologize for being a normal mammal. Elisa lives (and loves) with the brilliant and ruggedly handsome writer Edward Schwarzschild in Brooklyn and Albany, New York. Their baby son is likely to be utterly mortified by this book in about twelve years.

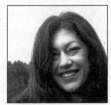

© Deb Stoner

J. A. K. Andres is a writer, educator, and counselor. She holds a B.A. in history from Yale and an M.S. in school counseling from Johns Hopkins. She lives in Portland, Oregon, and currently juggles four screenplays, three children, two dogs, and one hunk of a man.

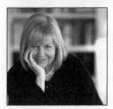

© Jill Posener

Susie Bright is a feminist sex critic and erotic educator. Author of bestselling books *Full Exposure* and *The Sexual State of the Union,* cofounder of On Our Backs, her new memoir is *Big Sex Little Death* (Seal Press). Visit her at www.susiebright.com.

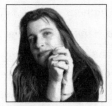

© Michael Falco

Susan Cheever is the bestselling author of twelve books, including *Louisa May Alcott: A Personal Biography,* five novels, and two memoirs. As a bestselling novelist and biographer, who garnered critical and popular accolades for *Home Before Dark,* her account of her father, novelist John Cheever's life, she appreciates intimately what it means to grow up immersed in the world of letters and under the implacable influence of an iconoclastic parent. And, of course, she knows well the challenges faced by a modern woman seeking fulfillment from and balance among the multiple facets of a complicated life. Her work has been nominated for the National Book Critics Circle Award and won the *Boston Globe* Winship Medal. She lives in New York City.

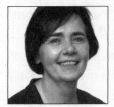

Courtesy of the *New York Times*

Gail Collins is an op-ed columnist for the *New York Times*. She has also served as the *Times* editorial page editor —the first woman ever to hold the post. She is the author of four books, including two histories of women in America. Ms. Collins began her journalistic career in Connecticut, where she founded the Connecticut State News Bureau (CSNB), which provided coverage of the state capitol to daily and weekly newspapers. When she sold it in 1977, the CSNB was the largest news service of its kind in the country, with more than thirty newspaper clients. She then moved to New York, where she worked at a number of news organizations and was a columnist for *New York Newsday* and the *New York Daily News*. Ms. Collins's latest book, *When Everything Changed*, is a history of American women since 1960. She is also the author of *America's Women: 400 Years of Dolls, Drudges, Helpmates and Heroines; Scorpion Tongues*, a history of gossip and American politics, and *The Millennium Book*, which she cowrote with her husband, Dan Collins. Ms. Collins grew up attending Catholic school, and in this piece she reflects on how human sexuality was (and wasn't) introduced in the classroom.

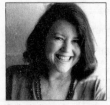
© Jim Holmes

Rosemary Daniell decided early in her writing life to break the two taboos with which she had been brought up as a southern woman—never to speak openly of anger or sexuality. Her beautiful, talented mother's suicide had shown her where such repression led, and truth telling became Rosemary's imperative, resulting in such controversial books as her first collection of poems, *A Sexual Tour of the Deep South*, and her memoirs, *Fatal Flowers: On Sin, Sex, and Suicide in the Deep South* and *Sleeping with Soldiers: In Search of the Macho Man*, both forerunners of the current memoir trend. Her most recent books are *Secrets of the Zona Rosa: How Writing (and Sisterhood) Can Change Women's Lives* and *Confessions of a (Female) Chauvinist;* she is the author of three other books of poetry and prose. Among her awards are two National Endowment grants in Literature—one in poetry, another in fiction. Known as one of the best writing coaches in the country, Rosemary is also the founder of Zona Rosa, the series of writing-and-living workshops for women she leads throughout the country and in Europe. She is profiled in the book *Feminists Who*

Changed America, 1963–1975; in 2008, she received a Governor's Award in the Humanities for her impact on the state of Georgia.

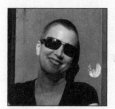
© Paula Allen

Eve Ensler is a playwright, performer, and activist. She is the award-winning author of *The Vagina Monologues,* which has been published in forty-eight languages and performed in over 140 countries. Eve's other works include *Necessary Targets, The Treatment, The Good Body, Insecure At Last: A Political Memoir,* and *I Am an Emotional Creature: The Secret Life of Girls Around the World.* Eve has written for the *Washington Post,* the *Guardian, Glamour, Huffington Post,* and *O, the Oprah Magazine.* She is the founder of V-Day, the global activist movement to end violence against women and girls, which has raised over $80 million for grassroots groups working to end violence against women and girls. Eve was named one of *US News & World Report'*s "Best Leaders" in association with the Center for Public Leadership (CPL) at Harvard Kennedy School, and is the recipient of a Guggenheim Fellowship in Playwriting and an Obie Award.

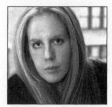
© Ben Ritter

Molly Jong-Fast wrote about her wild life as a girl in 1990s New York in a novel, *Normal Girl,* and a memoir, *Girl [Maladjusted].* Her third book, *The Social Climber's Handbook,* came out in April 2011 from Villard/Random House. She lives in New York City with her three children and two lizards, and her husband who does not like to be written about, at all, ever.

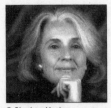

© Stephen Mosher

Susan Kinsolving is a poet and the recipient of four international fellowships, which were frustratingly awarded without a fine foreign fellow. Her books are: *The White Eyelash, Among Flowers, Dailies & Rushes,* a finalist for The National Book Critics Circle Award, and forthcoming *My Glass Eye.* (Forthcoming is not a pun.) Kinsolving teaches poetry and prudery in The Bennington Writing Seminars.

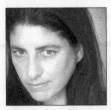

© Gabrielle Revere

Julie Klam is the author of a memoir, *Please Excuse My Daughter,* and the *New York Times* bestseller *You Had Me at Woof: How Dogs Taught Me the Secrets of Happiness.* She writes for *O, the Oprah Magazine, Glamour, Harper's Bazaar,* and the *New York Times Magazine.* She lives in New York City with her husband, her daughter, too many dogs, and a lot of turtlenecks.

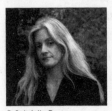

© Timothy Saccenti

Jean Hanff Korelitz is a native New Yorker currently in exile in New Jersey. She is the author of four novels, including *Admission* and *The White Rose,* a novel for children and a collection of poems, and a contributor to many magazines, including *Vogue* and *More.*

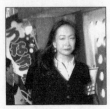

© Kerry Raftis

After **Min Jin Lee**'s husband, Christopher, recovered from the shock that she would not be writing about him (alone) for this compelling volume about sex, she decided that it might be safe to contribute an essay after all, since her mother and father would likely never learn about it. It also occurred to her that one day her son, Sam, might think she was far more interesting (read cooler) than she appeared. Lee is the author of the novel *Free Food for Millionaires,* which was a number one Book Sense Pick, a *New York Times* Editors' Choice, a *Wall Street Journal* Juggle Book Club selection, and a national bestseller. It was a "Top Ten Novels of the Year" for the *Times* of London, NPR'S *Fresh Air,* and *USA Today.* Her essays have appeared in the *Wall Street Journal, Travel + Leisure, Food & Wine, Vogue, Condé Nast Traveler,* and the *Times* of London. She was a columnist for the *Chosun Ilbo.* Lee lives in Tokyo with her husband and son.

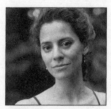
© Thad Russell

Ariel Levy is a staff writer at the *New Yorker* magazine, where she writes frequently about sexuality and gender. She has profiled the radical feminist Andrea Dworkin, the intersex South African runner Caster Semenya, and the lesbian separatist Lamar Van Dyke. Levy is also the author of *Female Chauvinist Pigs: Women and the Rise of Raunch Culture.* Her work has been anthologized in *The Best American Essays* and *The Best American Crime Reporting.*

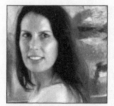
© Daniel Garvin

Margot Magowan has been trying to save the world since she was nine years old when a random woman in San Francisco offered her a picket sign and some free candy. Margot grew up to cofound the Woodhull Institute, an organization that trains women leaders and change makers. Today Margot can be found blogging or speaking about issues that affect women. She's appeared on TV and radio programs including CNN, *Good Morning America*, Fox News, and MSNBC; her articles have been in *Glamour, Salon,* the *San Jose Mercury News,* and other newspapers; her blog, Reel-Girl, rates media and products on girl empowerment. Now, living with her husband and three small kids, Margot would be perfectly happy to stop arguing with everyone about everything and only write fiction.

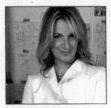

© Jeremy Balderson

Marisa Acocella Marchetto is a cartoonista/ activista and the author of the graphic memoir *Cancer Vixen* (Knopf), which she is adapting into a movie starring Cate Blanchett. She is a contributor to the *New Yorker,* and has been published in the *New York Times, Glamour, Elle, Bon Appétit, Harper's Bazaar, O, the Oprah Magazine, ESPN Magazine,* and the *Observer* (UK). As an activista, she has helped raise over a million dollars for the Breast Cancer Research Foundation and has raised a half million dollars for the Cancer Vixen Fund, which funds free breast screenings for women who are uninsured. Presently Marisa is finishing her graphic novel and is chained to her drawing board.

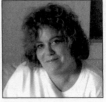

© Zoë Merkin-Brod

Daphne Merkin is a cultural critic who has made a name for herself with her often unnerving candor and elegantly High/Low reflections on issues of family, religion, depression, psychotherapy, and sex. She is a contributing writer for the *New York Times Magazine* and was previously a staff writer for the *New Yorker* for five years. She has also contributed to a wide variety of other publications, including the *New York Times Book Review, Vogue, Elle, Travel & Leisure, Allure, Slate,* the *Daily Beast,* and *Bookforum.* She has taught courses on the art of reading and creative nonfiction at the 92nd Street Y and Marymount College. Ms. Merkin is the author of two books: an autobiographical novel, *Enchantment,* and *Dreaming of Hitler,* a collection of essays. She is currently at work on a memoir about chronic depression, tentatively titled *The Black Season.* She lives in New York City with her daughter.

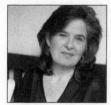

© The Estate of Inge Morath
at Magnum Photos

Honor Moore's poetry collections are *Red Shoes, Darling,* and *Memoir,* and she is the author of *The Bishop's Daughter,* a memoir, and *The White Blackbird,* a life of her grandmother, the painter Margarett Sargent—both now available in paperback.

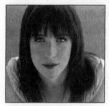

© Sarah Shatz

Meghan O'Rourke is the author of *The Long Goodbye,* a memoir about grief; and the poetry collections *Halflife* (W. W. Norton), which was a finalist for the Forward First Book Prize, and *Once,* forthcoming in 2011. A culture critic for *Slate,* she has published essays and poetry in the *New Yorker,* the *Nation, Poetry,* and elsewhere, and has written frequently about the cultural anxiety surrounding women's sexual freedom.

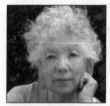

© Courtesy of the Roiphe
family

Anne Roiphe has written eighteen books and enough articles to sink a small life raft. Now in her seventies, she is coming to the end of the story, which her children and grandchildren will continue. Body to body they were made and body to body they will make others in their image and she can't think of a finer way to pass our time on earth.

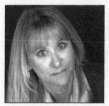

© Todd Rafalovich

Linda Gray Sexton is the author of the memoir *Half in Love: Surviving the Legacy of Suicide,* published by Counterpoint Press, as well as four novels. Her first critically acclaimed memoir, *Searching for Mercy Street: My Journey Back to My Mother, Anne Sexton,* will be reissued by Couterpoint in April 2011. She lives in California with her husband, her two sons, and her dalmatian, Breeze.

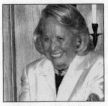

© Courtesy of Liz Smith

Liz Smith calls herself "the two-thousand-year-old gossip columnist." Arriving in Manhattan from the University of Texas journalism school in 1949, she has worked in celebrity/showbiz for fifty-seven years. She has written for seven different New York City newspapers and for almost every magazine. She was a CBS radio producer for Mike Wallace, then an NBC-TV producer in the fifties. Later, she went on camera at NBC and won an Emmy for reporting from the battleship *Intrepid* on the fortieth anniversary of World War II. In her bestselling memoir *Natural Blonde,* she wrote about being a war bride.

She appears on Fox News and in seventy newspapers. She has become a voice of reason and common sense, observing popular culture. Her philanthropy is legend—raising millions for AIDS research, Literacy Partners, New York Restoration Project, the Police Athletic League, the Mayor's Fund to Advance New York, and the New York Landmarks Conservancy. (They made her a "Living Landmark" in 1996.)

Liz is amused when dubbed "too nice." Says she, "If this is true, why did Frank Sinatra denounce me on world stages? Why did Donald Trump try to buy my newspaper so he could fire me? Why did P.R. flack Bobby Zarem say I'd had a woman killed? Why did Sean Connery want to stick my column where the sun don't shine? Why did Sean Penn run out of a building when we were introduced?"

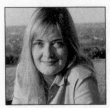

© Guy Tillim

Jann Turner is a writer and filmmaker. She is the author of the novels *Heartland* and *Southern Cross,* and the children's book *Home Is Where You Find It*. She's an award-winning filmmaker who has written and directed hundreds of hours of television, and she is the director of the feature films *White Wedding* and *Paradise Stop*.

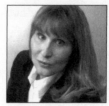

© Sigrid Estrada

Barbara Victor is a journalist who has covered the Middle East for most of her career. Based in Paris, she has worked for a variety of international magazines, newspapers, and television programs. She scored the first interview of Muammar Gaddafi after the November 1986 American bombardment of Libya and her interview was a cover story for *US News & World Report*. She is also the author of five novels, which have been translated into more than twenty-five languages, and nine nonfiction books, one of which, a biography of Hanan Ashrawi, was nominated for the 1995 Pulitzer Prize.

After living in Paris for twenty-two years, Barbara finally came home and married the man of her dreams. She lives in New York with her husband and three dogs, but still writes books, lectures on women's issues, and writes a blog entitled Mecca (see barbaravictor.com).

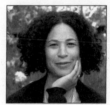

© David Fenton

Rebecca Walker is the author of the bestselling, award-winning memoirs *Black, White, and Jewish* and *Baby Love;* and editor of the anthologies *To Be Real, What Makes a Man,* and *One Big Happy Family.* She parents avidly, writes constantly, lectures widely, and teaches seminars on creative nonfiction and the art of memoir around the world.

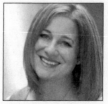

© Andrea Cipriani Mecchi

Jennifer Weiner was born in 1970 on an army base in Louisiana. She grew up in Connecticut, graduated with a degree in English literature from Princeton University, and worked as a newspaper reporter until the publication of her first book. She is the author of the novels *Good in Bed; In Her Shoes,* which was turned into a major motion picture; *Little Earthquakes; Goodnight Nobody;* the short story collection *The Guy Not Taken; Cer-*

tain Girls, the sequel to *Good in Bed; Best Friends Forever;* and *Fly Away Home.* There are more than eleven million copies of her books in print in thirty-six countries. She can be found on Facebook, on Twitter, and, in real life, in Philadelphia, where she lives with her family.

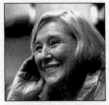

© Jonathan Dockar-Drysdale

Fay Weldon has been writing novels, stories, stage and screen plays for a good forty years and shows no sign of stopping. In Britain she is known as a national treasure, which she supposes to be better than being a national disgrace. She has been married three times and has four sons, three stepsons and one stepdaughter.

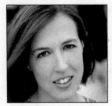

© Adrian Kinloch

Jessica Winter is a senior editor at *TIME.* Her writing has appeared in *Slate,* the *Boston Globe,* the *Los Angeles Times,* the *Believer,* and many other publications. She lives in Brooklyn.

About the Editor

Erica Jong is a poet, novelist, and essayist, best known for her eight *New York Times* bestselling novels: *Fear of Flying* (which has sold twenty-six million copies in more than forty languages); *How to Save Your Own Life;* *Fanny: Being the True History of the Adventures of Fanny Hackabout-Jones; Parachutes & Kisses; Shylock's Daughter (previously called Serenissima); Any Woman's Blues; Inventing Memory;* and *Sappho's Leap.*

© Mary Ellen Mark

Her midlife memoir, *Fear of Fifty,* remains a major international bestseller.

Ms. Jong is also the author of seven award-winning collections of poetry. Her latest, *Love Comes First,* was released by Tarcher-Penguin in January 2009.

Ms. Jong is also the author of several nonfiction books. Her work has appeared all over the world.

Known for her commitment to women's rights, copyright, and free expression, Ms. Jong is a frequent lecturer in the United States and abroad. She was president of the Authors Guild and now serves on its board.

She has established a program for young writers at her alma mater, Barnard College.

Columbia University (where she received her M.A. in eighteenth-century English literature) acquired her literary archive in 2008.

Ms. Jong has been honored with the United Nations Award for Excellence in Literature, *Poetry* magazine's Bess Hokin Prize, and the Deauville Award in France. In Italy, she has received the Sigmund Freud Award and the first Fernanda Pivano Prize, named for the woman who introduced Ernest Hemingway, Allen Ginsberg, and Erica Jong to Italy.

Ms. Jong is working on a novel featuring "a woman of a certain age."

Fear of Flying is in preparation as a BBC miniseries.

Sugar in My Bowl is her first anthology.

For more information, please visit her websites: www.ericajong .com and www.sugarinmybowl.com.